greater EXPECTATIONS

Living with Down syndrome in the 21st century

Jan Gothard

FOREWORD BY PROFESSOR FIONA STANLEY AC

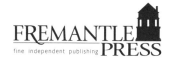

FREMANTLE PRESS
fine independent publishing

To my daughters Katie, Maddie and Erin

WELCOME
by Justin Marshall

I was asked to write something for this book because I know a lot about Down syndrome. That's because I have Down syndrome. I've had it for my whole life. I used to be angry about that and didn't think it was fair. But I'm used to it now and it doesn't bother me anymore.

When I was born the doctor told my mum and dad that I had Down syndrome straight away. He knew because he saw a straight line across my hand, stubby fingers, and when he picked me up I was floppy.

When I was two my sister Caroline was born, when I was five Juliet was born and when I was ten Sarah was born — now that's three sisters I have to cope with! But they are actually my best friends and they have always been proud of me.

I have had a go at lots of different things like any other boy. I used to call my mum a pushy mother but I was only joking. I used to go to Riding for the Disabled and Boy Scouts. I went to trampolining and drama classes, and I played tee-ball and football. I also had piano lessons for a while but chucked it in because I didn't like practising. I also belonged to a swimming club called the Superfins.

I went to Davallia Primary School then Christ Church Grammar School. I was in the Education Support Unit but went to some mainstream classes as well. In the junior school the boys sometimes teased me and called me names. I felt angry and sad and frustrated and sometimes I felt like crying. Sometimes when we went out people would stare at me because I look different. That made me angry and embarrassed. Sometimes people talked about me in front of me like I wasn't there, and I would be offended by that.

They think I'm not capable and that I don't understand what they are saying. They must think I'm stupid. Then they are surprised when they find out I know more than they do about rock music and Hollywood movies, and other interesting information which I've read on the internet and in the World Book Encyclopedia.

In my last year at school I gave a talk about what it's like to have Down syndrome. My teacher was very impressed and entered it in a creative writing competition run by the Down Syndrome Association. I was the winner and won a trophy. Since then I have given lots of talks. My mum and I have even been to Singapore for the World Down Syndrome Congress. I gave a speech to seven hundred people from thirty-five countries. I wasn't nervous, I was confident.

When I finished school I got a job at Westcare which is a printing company. I also went to TAFE. I catch the train by myself because I like being independent.

I walk to the gym near my house twice a week. I've been going there since I left school. I've got a personal trainer who makes me push my body. I was the WA Disabled Sports Association state powerlifting champion for four years.

When I joined a rowing club for disabled people called Freedom on the River I went to the National Rowing Championships in Victoria and Tasmania. Both times I won a gold medal. I felt good when everyone was shaking my hand and patting me on the back and saying 'Congratulations mate.' I was pleased with myself and was glad that I had given it my best shot.

I think it is hard for other people to understand what it's like to have Down syndrome. But I'm proud of myself because I'm smart and I can do things like anyone else.

This book is about people like me and my family. I hope you will like reading it.

contents

FOREWORD
by Fiona Stanley AC

One of the first things that struck me when I put down this book was the transformation through its pages of the families whose stories are told. From the first moment of stunned disbelief when they learn their new baby has Down syndrome and fear they are never going to be able to deal with raising their child, we watch parents coping with difficult social choices, and with the medical issues that sometimes accompany Down syndrome — and we see them learning to live with the challenges life has presented them.

Then at some point a corner is turned and parents become increasingly proactive: lobbying, fighting health providers and schools and government departments for the rights of their children, creating support groups, and organising the education and accommodation they want for their children. Having a child with Down syndrome certainly changes your life.

With this book Jan Gothard makes an important contribution to the literature on Down syndrome and on disability in general in the twenty-first century. The personal and autobiographical stories are set against a comprehensive account of the broader social and historical context of Down syndrome and of disability generally.

It is the book I'd want to read if I had had a child with Down syndrome. It's the book I'd recommend to parents who already have a child with Down syndrome, or for whom prenatal testing has indicated Down syndrome, and they are wondering what on earth the future holds. As a scientist working in the area of child health, I would also recommend it to all those people — teachers, health professionals including doctors, and policy makers — who work with people with disabilities or who make the decisions which affect them. Professional attitudes play an enormous role in shaping the lives of people with disabilities and their families, and this book gives a privileged insight into the impact of such decision-making, for better and worse, at a personal level.

What people need foremost is information. Reliable information. The more we know, the less foreign is the terrain and the better we can deal with the masses of misinformation that still abound. And, just as important, we need to know we are not alone, that others have faced the decisions and dilemmas that we are now facing. That our responses are not abnormal. *Greater Expectations* provides all this and more. It shows children, young people, men and women with Down syndrome, 'busy doing perfectly normal things, getting on with their lives.'

Some chapters will be confronting reading for any new parent, but the overriding feeling is deeply positive. In society at large, enormous progress has been made in the last few decades. The period when parents were encouraged to give their children over to institutions, encouraged to believe that their child was beyond schooling and was unlikely to live into adulthood is over — very largely thanks to the 'courage and stubborn persistence' of an older generation of parents of children with Down syndrome 'driven by love or duty to offer their children a better life.'

That better life — with opportunities in education, sport, play and work that were hardly dreamt of a generation ago — is here now, but there is still quite a way to go. As Jan Gothard reminds us, 'We owe all this to the parents who fought against negative expectations; we owe it to our children to keep our expectations growing.' This book will surely feed those greater expectations.

Professor Fiona Stanley AC, October 2010
Patron, Down Syndrome Association of Western Australia

PARTICIPANTS

The following people were interviewed or provided personal information for this project between 1996 and 2010. Mavis Simpson, Muriel Mann and Trish Weston were interviewed by Helen Robertson between 1992 and 1995; Trish Weston was subsequently reinterviewed. Real names are marked with an asterisk; all others are pseudonyms.

Alison Austen, mother of James
James Austen
Dirk Bakker, father of Amelia
Malcolm Barnes (email only)
Eddie Bartnik (Disability Services Commission)*
Wendy and Keith Brookton, parents of Mark
Heather Burton, mother of Lucy
Lucy Burton
Britt Canning, mother of Jack
Christine Conway
Andrew Danes, father of Cameron
Ana Diaz, mother of Benita
Benita Diaz
Cathy Donovan (Down Syndrome Association of
   Western Australia)*
Dr Luigi D'Orsogna*
Iris Fisher, grandmother of Trudy
Denise Flynn, sister of Frank
Diana Foster, mother of John
Pamela Franklin, mother of Catherine
Helen Golding, mother of Damian, Charlotte and Josie
Bernard Grant, father of Angus
Lisa Greenwood, mother of Gareth
Richard Gregson, father of Jordan
Gordon Griffith, carer of Richard Stevens
Eloise Hartley
Brenda Harvey, mother of Grace
Rhonda Henry, sister of Charlie King

Emily Howard, mother of Joseph
Geraldine Howe
Penny Innes, mother of Rebecca
Rebecca Innes
Nathan Johnson
Marg King, sister of Charlie King
Rachel Kingston
Anna Klein, mother of Michael
Michael Klein
Carol Lambert, mother of Malia
Karen Langley, mother of Shannon da Silva
Jude Lawrence, mother of Laura Middleton
Alex Major
Muriel and William Mann, parents of Geoffrey
Jill Mather, sister of Richard Stevens
Claudia Mansour, mother of Theresa
Laura Middleton
Luke Middleton, father of Laura
Loretta Muller, mother of Cameron Danes
Jennifer and Sunil Ravi, parents of Amber
Virginia and Alan Robb, parents of Georgia
Janet Rossi, mother of Sandra
Mavis Simpson, mother of Trevor
Jackie Softly (Down Syndrome Association of
    Western Australia)*
Richard Stevens
Adam Szabo
Mary Tanaka, mother of Lucas
Nicola Webb
Steph and Paul Webb, parents of Nicola
Ellen Wentworth
Leah Wentworth, mother of Ellen, mother-in-law of
    Adam Szabo
Trish Weston, mother of Will Weston
Jeremy Young

ACKNOWLEDGEMENTS

As an oral history, this book could not have been written without the readiness of individuals to open up their homes and hearts. Parents revealed their family lives to me with honesty and candour, while the unparalleled opportunity to interview people with Down syndrome was an enormous privilege. One of the reasons this book took me so long to write was my recognition that I had been entrusted with priceless sources, and the responsibility for shaping the material — other people's lives — was onerous. In the decade I spent researching and interviewing for this book I accrued great obligations to many people and I remain inspired by the stories I was told.

I would like to acknowledge and thank all the following for their contribution.

For a range of information on life with Down syndrome, suggestions and recollections: Caryl Baily, Rick Berg, Paul Brokenshire, Bronwyn Callaghan, Isabel Cardenosa, Margaret Cardenosa, Nick Cartmel, Anna Collis, Jenny Collis, Maria Crawford, Evelyn Daniels, Andrew Domahidy, Cathy Donovan, Stephen Donovan, Ian Duckham, Kiki Ekasasi, Sharon Ford, Charlie Fox, Chitto Ghosh, Margaret Gilham, Erin Gothard-Fox, Madeleine Gothard-Fox, Katie Gothard-Leigh, Andrea Griffiths-Ghosh, Jenny Guhl, Julia Hales, Kate Hall, Andrew Harcourt, Gina Harcourt, Alis Hart, Jonnine Hutton, Julie Ireland, Julie Jalawadi, Raj Jalawadi, Wendy Jones, Linda Katuna-Rich, Brian Kealy, Joanne Kent, Kay King, Peter Koenig, Ruth Koenig, Mary Lockyer, Donna Macale, Beth Marchbank, Lauren Marchbank, Margaret Marshall, Lisa Martin, Al Mason, Sharon Mason, Katherine Matsumoto, Monica McGillivray, Stephen McEwen, Judith Mincham, Lillian Mincham, Alice Mourad, Danika Newton, Maureen Newton,

Phil Newton, Cy Payne, Olive Price, Val Ricciardo, Marcia Rowlands, Charles Ryder, Sabine Schreuder, David Shields, Jackie Softly, Maida Stern, Walter Stern, Nichola Wood and Stefan Zwickl.

For advice on statistics and information from their own professional fields, I thank Cathie Clement; Luigi D'Orsogna; Barry Quinn; Sylvie St-Jacques; Eddie Bartnik, Disability Services Commission; Angie Godden, Mid West Community Living Association Inc.; Jenny Bourke, Telethon Institute for Child Health Research; Leath Merton, Western Diagnostic Pathology; Sue Robertson, EDGE Employment; and Carol Bower, Natasha Nassar and Edwina Rudy, Birth Defects Registry, King Edward Memorial Hospital.

Bill Bunbury, David Leach, Tim Fetherstonhaugh, Lois Gothard, Virginia Rowland and Nichola Wood offered feedback on various chapters and drafts; and I am also grateful for the support of colleagues Helen Brash and Jean Chetkovich.

David Guhl gave enthusiastic permission to use his painting for the cover; Justin Marshall provided first-hand reflections on Down syndrome. Mona Neumann was the photographer of the DSAWA 'Beyond the Myths' exhibition, photos from which appear in this book. The cartoon 'It's Sue actually' appears with permission of artist Simon Kneebone, and the figure on page 83 is used with the permission of author Carol Bower of the Birth Defects Registry.

Helen Robertson, formerly of Activ Foundation Inc., conducted three earlier interviews which I drew on in writing this book. Anne Atkinson interviewed me, and she and Maryon Allbrook both gave early support and advice.

Anne McBride, Heather Campbell and Genelle Jones combined transcribing and administrative assistance with a real commitment to this project.

A Community History grant from Lotterywest enabled me to interview families in regional Western Australia, to pay for transcribing and to extend the scope of the project well beyond my earliest plans.

Staff at Fremantle Press were wonderful: Clive Newman and Ray Coffey with their initial enthusiasm for this book; Jane Fraser who oversaw the publication, with assistance from Naama Amram; and Janet Blagg, my editor. It was a privilege to work with Janet again. I particularly thank the Press for its professionalism and patience.

The Down Syndrome Association of Western Australia (DSAWA) supported this project from the very outset. Though it grew well beyond what any of us had envisaged and took far longer to complete, the Association retained an unflagging belief that the book would eventually see daylight. Many of the people interviewed for the book are Association members. Special thanks go to Association staff Cathy Donovan, Julie Ireland and Jackie Softly for reading the manuscript, to Carol Manus for pulling out resources from the DSAWA library for me, and to the Committee for financial support with transcribing. Of course, views presented in this book are mine alone and should not be taken as representing the views of the DSAWA.

The book was inspired by my three daughters — Katie, Maddie and Erin — and it is a record of a defining element in their lives. And finally, to my partner Charlie Fox. Always a staunch believer in my capacity to get this book written, he carved out time from our family budget to enable me to finish it, read drafts, and provided continuing scholarly advice on many aspects of the history of disability in Western Australia. It certainly helps living with an expert! Charlie has been with me on every step of this journey, which began long before I ever thought about mapping it in a book.

Jan Gothard

INTRODUCTION

Born in Western Australia in 1977, Christopher Derkacz had Down syndrome. As sometimes happened to children like him in the 1970s, his family relinquished him, he was made a ward of the state and put into care. In January 1979, when he was just twenty-three months old, his foster mother took him to Perth's Princess Margaret Hospital for Children, suffering from croup. She thought she had left him in the best place and the safest hands, but she was wrong. Christopher had a further attack of croup that night but, instead of reviving him, the nursing staff left him to die, because the notes prepared by his doctor were marked: 'Not for resuscitation — no cardiac massage or intubation.'[1] At the inquest, the nurses who had attended Christopher were advised not to give evidence, on the grounds that it might incriminate them; but, according to both the press report and a subsequent question raised in the Western Australian parliament, the doctor in charge of the case said that children like Christopher should not even be admitted into the hospital's intensive care unit, and that if they lived they too often became a social burden.

Australians are not the only people who have refused appropriate medical treatment to people with disabilities like Down syndrome. There have been celebrated cases in both the United States and the United Kingdom of individuals fighting, usually unsuccessfully, for the right even to go on a transplant waiting list. After a much publicised campaign in the mid 1990s, American woman Sandra Jensen finally received a heart and lung transplant, though she died from complications sixteen months later. She was almost certainly the first person with Down syndrome, and may well be the only such individual to date, to have received a major organ transplant.[2] But while progress has not always been straightforward, I believe we have come a long way from that moment in January 1979 when a toddler was refused life-saving treatment for an everyday childhood ailment like croup, because a doctor decided that a life with Down syndrome simply wasn't worth living.

This book is not about Christopher and Sandra, but it is about people like them, and their families. It's also about a community. From the day my daughter Madeleine was born in 1992, I have been part of a community which stretches across state and national boundaries, overriding language, race and ethnicity. I have been approached by a Chinese-American family in the Te Papa museum in Wellington, New Zealand who, after a few penetrating glances, wandered over to ask how my daughter was going. Two of my daughters were with me, but I had no doubt which one they meant. I have exchanged smiles with a Korean couple in Cambodia, members of a tour group, as they and their adolescent son explored the Khmer ruins at Angkor. My partner Charlie and I have been known to stare as we drive past an individual on the street, or when we spot a family on the beach or at a shopping centre — are they too part of our 'community'? I once resisted the temptation to stalk a young woman wearing a staff uniform in a hospital corridor, intensely curious to know exactly how she was employed there and whether they had room for another one. We have been approached more than once in coffee shops and parks by parents and grandparents who have remarked on our 'lovely family'. We were out doing normal things, behaving in entirely usual and not always perfect ways, yet the phrase and compliment are always loaded with meaning. The day before my daughter was born, these people would have remained largely invisible to me, and my family to them.

'Community' can be purchased cheaply these days; for the price of a car sticker, anyone can attest that they are friends of the ABC or that their 'other family' is the East Fremantle Yacht Club. Members of what I think of as the Down syndrome community, and the disability community more generally, may share nothing more than a familiarity with disability and no doubt many would rather share less. For writer Kathy Evans, the public recognition of her daughter's 'community membership' was no 'warm and fuzzy moment'.

> It served only as a reminder that my child was not just a member of my family, built from the atoms of generations of Celtic ancestors, but part of a distinctly recognizable breed, like poodles or Siamese cats.[3]

Questions about what it means to have Down syndrome in the family, how individuals and families experience that situation, and the social implications of living within that 'community' are contentious. Brian Stratford, doyen of the Down syndrome world, has written glowingly of the community in terms of parent organisations across the world which contain within them otherwise warring parties, bound together by the common cause of improving the lot of their kids. He writes of a variety of such bodies, including 'Catholics and protestants in Northern Ireland ... work[ing] together towards the development of their children with Down's syndrome,' the Indian Down syndrome association with its multi-religious membership, and the Zimbabwean association comprising 'both black and white, taking into consideration only the needs of their children and their support for each other,' and concludes that: 'John Langdon Down has given his name not only to a single pathological condition causing mental handicap, but to a worldwide community of people with potential.[4] I am less sanguine than Stratford about the potential for harmony within the Down syndrome community, but less defensive than Evans. This book explores what I consider to be the transcending experience of living with Down syndrome; but it does so in full recognition that, like most communities, the differences within it may be as great as the factors that create it.

Once, a child with a difference was a child to be hidden or denied, but since perhaps the 1950s, as institutionalisation of children with disabilities began to be questioned by professionals and, increasingly, by parents, so too writing about a child with a physical or intellectual disability has developed into an autobiographical genre. One of the first people to publish a book in English about their experiences was singer/songwriter and actor Dale Evans. In 1950, she and her husband, renowned stage cowboy Roy Rogers, became the parents of Robin Elizabeth, who had Down syndrome and who died just short of her second birthday. *Angel Unaware* is written in the voice of baby Robin, cast as an angel sent to earth to spread joy and awareness. The book, motivated by the couple's Christian beliefs, was published only with difficulty — it was not a popular topic at that time. However, as one of the earliest of such 'true confessional' works, the book gave hope to many who read it and has sold over a million copies. In 2004 a fiftieth anniversary edition was published.

Is it easier or harder for families of note to accept their difference? Anne de Gaulle was the daughter of General Charles de Gaulle and his wife Yvonne. Born in 1928 with Down syndrome, she was never separated from the rest of the family and lived a fully included life, her acceptance and protection part of the family's deeply held values. Her death in 1948 left the general devastated.[5] On the other hand, playwright

Arthur Miller's son Daniel, born with Down syndrome in 1966, was institutionalised at birth, despite the wishes of the boy's mother, Inge Morath, who continued to visit him throughout his life. Though Miller did not mention this son in his autobiography, he was apparently reconciled with him later in life when Daniel left the institution, and shortly before the playwright's death, Miller bequeathed Daniel, along with his siblings, an equal share of his assets.[6]

It took Pulitzer and Nobel Prize winning author Pearl S. Buck thirty years to publicly promote knowledge of her much-loved daughter. Born in 1920, Carol was 'mentally retarded', institutionalised from adolescence and thereafter kept out of the public gaze. Buck's book about Carol, *The Child Who Never Grew* (1950), was re-published in 1992, and as the foreword notes:

> For families whose lives were haunted by the sad mystery of mental retardation, all the scientific explanations in the world would not have as much impact as a famous, respected person disclosing publicly, 'I speak as one who knows.'

Perceptively, referring to the courage it took to self-reveal in the 1950s, the foreword also refers to 'the 1990s' tell-all atmosphere of celebrities baring their most private scars.' Whereas having a child with a disability makes most people feel uncomfortably 'different', it somehow seems to give celebrities a veneer of normality by showing that, just like the rest of us, the beautiful people too can experience life's challenges. For that reason, the birth of a child with a disability is often an occasion for the media to descend. Yet the publicity can also become an important and uplifting focus for more 'regular' families, and there is no doubt that giving disability more currency can serve valuable political ends, with disability societies around the world quick to acknowledge or seize the patronage of celebrities such as racing car driver Damon Hill or rock star Nik Kershaw, both of whom have a child with Down syndrome.

The birth of Domenica Lawson in 1995 gave the Down syndrome community in Britain a powerful public voice through her father Dominic Lawson, former long-time editor of the London *Sunday Telegraph*, and her mother Rosa Monckton. Godmother Diana, Princess of Wales, added further cachet to Domenica's life, although we have not yet seen Domenica appear on television with kitchen goddess aunt Nigella Lawson. Since Domenica's birth, her parents have become highly articulate and outspoken critics of policies such as the assumption of automatic termination of Down syndrome pregnancies and both have written movingly about their rather different responses to their daughter's birth. Just as the death of the Princess of Wales raised awareness about wearing seatbelts and Kylie Minogue's breast cancer led to a rise in mammograms, the well-publicised birth of a child with Down syndrome in a prominent family sends out a message that this can happen to anyone. While it may also have increased the incidence of prenatal screening, the birth of Domenica Lawson underlined the fact that having a child with Down syndrome is not automatically such a bad thing.

That is, after all, the message which permeates auto-biographical accounts of living with a child with Down syndrome. Books and TV series with titles such as *Life Goes On* stress the continuities of existence after the arrival of a child with a difference. Michael Bérubé's wonderful *Life As We Know It* is an example of this genre, with Bérubé's son Jamie at the heart of the family, but alongside and taking up no more and no less space than Jamie's elder brother Nick. Nowadays too, there is a gratifying trend away from the beatification approach exemplified in *Angel Unaware*, which left many parents of less than saintly children a little uncomfortable; although the autobiographical *Expecting Adam* — with its blunt allusion to the supernatural guiding powers of the child with Down syndrome, even *in utero* — is clearly part of that older tradition. Despite their differences, however, what all these books reveal is that, as individuals, people have felt compelled to talk about the profound impact of the birth of a child with disability. Their powerful need to articulate their shock and reaction speaks volumes of the still-hidden nature of disability in society today.

Until recently, intellectual disability was a relatively unexplored theme in social and historical research in Australia, but over the past decade or so more has been written as disability has become an increasingly acknowledged dimension of social difference. This book represents a convergence of two streams of writing: personal and autobiographical parental accounts, and historical and contemporary analysis of disability. It ranges over themes associated with rites of passage and pivotal social moments and discusses birth experience and the acceptance of disability; family and community support; health issues; education; growing up and finding work, and independent living. All these themes are located within a broader social and historical context. The book also looks at family decision-making: continuing or terminating pregnancies; accepting or relinquishing children at birth, and learning how to let them go. Where possible, these themes are explored from the point of view of individuals with Down syndrome, as well as their families.

This book is based on more than sixty personal interviews recorded across Western Australia but it has broad geographical and social application beyond Australia, and certainly reinforces an understanding of the universalising aspects of some experiences of disability. Western Australia in fact has much to offer as a place to locate a study such as this because of the richness of the research already undertaken into disability and Down syndrome in this state. The 1996 edited collection *Under Blue Skies: The Social Construction of Intellectual Disability in Western Australia* is a pioneering history of intellectual disability in Western Australia and still remains unmatched by publications in other Australian states. Western Australia is also the home of the acclaimed Telethon Institute for Child Health Research whose director Professor Fiona Stanley is Patron of the Down Syndrome Association of Western Australia. The Telethon Institute has been responsible for producing a huge body of research data on issues such as the health and longevity of people with Down syndrome and the impact of prenatal screening. It also produced the *Down Syndrome Needs Opinions Wishes Study Report* in 2007, which surveyed more than three hundred Western Australian families living with Down syndrome. These and other publications have been used to complement the personal accounts in the pages which follow.

The people I interviewed were culturally and socially diverse and included Aboriginal and migrant families. I started interviewing more than a decade ago, which has given me the unexpected opportunity to revisit some of the earliest informants, in what eventually became an unplanned longitudinal study.[7] In the course of talking to people, it soon became apparent that the biggest factors determining one's experience of Down syndrome were place of residence — metropolitan or regional — and the era when an individual with Down syndrome was born. Services undreamt of in regional settings were often delivered to the doorstep in metropolitan Perth, while predictably, services waxed and waned and educational opportunities differed as state government policies shifted over time. More important for me than charting changes in policies and provision of services though, was finding out how people had responded to the opportunities available and how the choices they made affected their lives.

The majority of my interviews have been with parents, primarily mothers, and other carers of people with Down syndrome, but about one-third of the people I interviewed had Down syndrome. When I commenced interviewing, I wanted to focus very much on the question of what it meant to have Down syndrome, and I approached this issue in the broader context of finding out how young adults with Down syndrome lived their lives. What I found was how very like, in many ways, were the lives of the people I spoke to, compared to those of their peers who did not have a disability. Ranging in age from sixteen to their thirties when I interviewed them, the majority of those young adults lived at home with their parents. One young woman had taken out a mortgage and was buying her own home, a unit she shared with a friend who also had Down syndrome. Another man rented a unit in Fremantle where he lived by himself. One couple was married and living independently in a larger south-west town. None was in any form of residential facility, and none had been institutionalised at birth, which would have been more typical of older people with Down syndrome. Social interaction, recreation, education and training, relationships, work and family were the main focus of their lives and, while some clear differences existed — largely associated with independence — my interviews reinforced Jan Walmsley's observation that 'being a person with a learning disability is most akin to being a human being.'[8]

Sometimes documenting the normal can be difficult. The discrepancy between experiencing Down syndrome as 'normality', and living alongside it as a disability, is a profound one and, in trying to present different understandings of what it's like living with Down syndrome, one that I needed to keep very much in mind. My own experience of disability, and the experiences related to me by the carers and parents I interviewed, confirmed for me that disability can profoundly affect one's life. So while this book is based on optimism about the future and an overwhelming belief that people with disabilities such as Down syndrome can, should, and do lead normal lives, it is underpinned by a historian's awareness of past struggles to bring about change.

A researcher's position is never neutral, but I have felt particularly challenged by this work. My interest in disability is precisely as old as my daughter. As she has grown up I have become increasingly aware of how an everyday life lived with disability can be a political and social battleground, one of which my daughter still remains largely unaware but one in which her parents engage on a daily basis. I have experienced disability as both oppressive and 'disabling' and, as an interviewer, I always kept that in mind. I have much in common with many of the parents interviewed in terms of experiences associated with the recognition of a child's disability and working through the consequences, but many parents do not share my view of disability as a condition made worse by, but which could be made better by, social attitudes. This is a difficult line to tread but, as interviewer, I attempted to render my personal views invisible in the interviewing situation. My intention was, after all, to see how a range of people experience living with a disability, not to proselytise or see how many people shared my point of view. Clearly however, interviewing from within a community presents a number of challenges.[9] The Down syndrome community in Western Australia is a reasonably small one and as an interviewer

I always identified myself as a parent of a child with Down syndrome, believing that the informants' awareness that I too had 'been there', in fact still 'was there', could encourage the sharing of deeply-buried and sometimes painful memories. It was also a good starting point for interviews with people with Down syndrome too, explaining that I wanted to ask about their lives and, incidentally, about having Down syndrome, because of my daughter.

Equally challenging has been the question of how to use my own voice. I am an interviewer and researcher, but I too have a story to tell. The question of selecting interview extracts, locating them within the text, and above all, giving them weight, was a difficult one. The responsibility for interviewing, editing and writing was mine. However, in order to give my voice what I hope is no more than equal weighting with other parent voices, I primed a friend to interview me. Like all the other interviews in this book, that one too is used anonymously, and enables me to have 'my' voice heard directly.[10] I cannot deny though that as editor I have had the opportunity to select material and to stage manage to produce effects which suit my own convictions. As historian Ann Curthoys has noted of a similar challenge — writing a historical account of an episode in which she herself was a participant — 'Even if I satisfy myself that I have avoided these traps, will others believe that I have?'[11] I have to hope so. This book is not intended to fit into that autobiographical self-revelatory genre of books about how one family lives with disability; rather, it draws on multiple voices to show the plurality of that experience.

Interviewing people with an intellectual disability undoubtedly raises profound ethical questions for a researcher. As an interviewer and as someone who has been involved with disability for many years, I am well aware of the tendency identified by Karen Hirsch of speaking on behalf of people with disabilities, especially, as in this case, intellectual disability, and I took on board her caution that 'it is hard to overstate how resistant and pervasive is the cultural assumption that people with disabilities cannot speak for themselves.'[12] Among people with Down syndrome there are many who are more than capable of doing so, of telling an interviewer about the lives they lead, their experiences, interests and aspirations. More generally, in terms of self-expression, there are books authored by people with Down syndrome, ranging from the classic 1967 publication Nigel Hunt's *The World of Nigel Hunt* to Kingsley and Levitz's *Count Us In*, now in its second edition in 2007. Australian actor and advocate Ruth Cromer and young American advocate Karen Gaffney are both renowned speakers at international disability forums; in Western Australia, Justin Marshall is a frequent speaker on the topic of having Down syndrome. Such individuals, though, remain a tiny minority. While people with Down syndrome are not all similarly disabled, nor are they equally 'able'. Some people with Down syndrome are simply not articulate and to interview only those who could sustain a lucid conversation would be to misrepresent the community. As Brian Stratford observes,

> it is distressing for parents of a good number of children with Down's syndrome to be constantly hearing of near normal development and of high individual achievement when their own child is not making anything like that kind of progress.[13]

On that basis, one of the dilemmas I faced in undertaking this research project was balancing my desire to interview the most articulate people with Down syndrome I could find, with the recognition that other people's stories, less clearly verbalised and sometimes harder to render meaningful for an audience, were just as valid and perhaps more 'typical'. As an interviewer, I had more 'success' — in terms of lengthier and more in-depth interviews — with individuals who were more vocal, and whose interviews resulted in material which I was able to incorporate fairly directly into my text. But an interview program which focused only on the most successful or the most articulate individual would neglect many of the realities of living with Down syndrome. Other approaches, based on interviewing models employed by other researchers,[14] encouraged me to recognise that the end result of an interview should be more than just a recorded hour of lucid conversation or a flowing transcript. Instead of taking the informant's words directly, as one would usually do after an interview, as a researcher I have tried to take the meaning gleaned from each 'yes,' 'no' or silence, in conjunction with material from other sources such as parent interviews to create an indirect but meaningful narrative about individual lives. Thus, I see the role of the interviewer/editor and historian not as disempowering, because it detracts from the authority of the informant, but as enabling. The alternative, for less articulate people with intellectual disabilities, may well be silence.

In writing this book, I have tried to keep two themes in mind. The first is the role of parents in fighting for the advancement of their children. So many of the opportunities enjoyed by people of my daughter's generation and younger have come about because of the courage and stubborn persistence of an earlier generation of parents. In some cases, they had extremely limited expectations about their kids' capacities, having been told often enough by professionals that their kids had none. Nonetheless they persevered, driven by love or duty to offer their children a better life. Today parents are no longer handicapped by the belief that their children are beyond aid and as a result of the efforts of those earlier parents and far-sighted professionals, and of ideological shifts in understandings about disability, we now understand and act on the belief that people with disabilities have a potential which can be tapped and nurtured.

The second theme is belonging and inclusion. Support is increasingly there to assist people with disabilities to engage more fully in the community but it's still a journey down a one-way street. The state of full inclusion could be reached a lot more quickly, and would appear a lot more attractive to those who are still wary of it, if the rest of the community would meet people with disabilities halfway. Inclusion means more than simply having people with disabilities in mainstream classrooms and workplaces. It's about a state of mind which sees people with disabilities accepted as valued, significant and worthwhile members of society: people who have every right to belong. Though we have travelled light years in the past few decades, the absence of this mindset is unfortunately still evident in Australian society today, in places as far apart as maternity wards and the government's department of immigration.

Above all though I have kept in mind the profound changes that have occurred in the lives of people with Down syndrome, which make the story of Christopher Derkacz so confronting to us today. Consider people like Yolanda, Stefan and Judith, Nick, and countless others. Yolanda Berg is a member of the Western Australian government's Ministerial Advisory Council on Disability, contributing the critically important perspective of people living with intellectual disabilities to that forum. Linda Katuna Rich has worked with Coles Supermarkets since 1997, while Nick Cartmel has been employed at what is now the Western Australian state government's Disability Services Commission since 1992. Judith Mincham and Stefan Zwickl, who both have Down syndrome, got married in 2009. Samala Ghosh has won a prize for art in an open competition. Tom Softly flies with his father in a small plane and has medals for motorbike trials. Since 2007, Stephen Donovan has broken twelve world Down syndrome swimming records. Patrick Ricciardo has competed in the Rottnest Island swim. Julia Hales performed in her own show, *Soapy Dreaming*, in an acclaimed Solo Spot drama festival in 2008. Whether it's learning to read and write, ride a bike, catch a bus, hold down a job or, like Karen Gaffney, swim the English Channel, people with Down syndrome are doing it. Fifty years ago, they weren't. We owe all this to the parents who fought against negative expectations; we owe it to our children to keep our expectations growing.

Finally, I want to start this book by recalling my partner Charlie's words about our daughter Maddie.

When she turned one, we all got round to celebrate her birthday and thought back to the day she was born, all the tears, all the trauma, and I just couldn't help thinking, what on earth was all the fuss about?

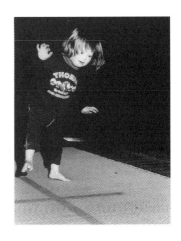

chapter 1

'THE BABY I'D DREAMED OF HAVING'

'I remember one of the nurses coming in and saying, "Well you're lucky she wasn't born thirty years ago, because she would have been put away and what have you. She'll go to school and she'll learn to read." I was lying there thinking, yes, but she was going to be a brain surgeon.'
(Heather Burton)

In 1990, two years before my daughter Madeleine was born, Fay Weldon's book *Darcy's Utopia* was published.

I think about my friend Erin as I often do. She has a Down's syndrome baby. We all knew it would be disastrous; we foretold that her husband would walk out, that her other children would suffer: we saw she was the only one of the family unit who couldn't bear not to see the fruit of her womb, however sour, ripen, drop and live. And that's how it turned out: the child, now twelve, is badly retarded. Erin is no more than its nurse; she manages without a husband, her other children are spiteful and embarrassed. Erin talks about the joy the mindless child brings her — well, so it may, but her love for it has been most destructive for others. Left to us, friends and family, we would have said no, Erin, sorry, not for you. This baby you insist on having keeps other babies out, ones which won't cause this distress to you and yours. Just not this one; Erin, try again.[15]

Images of the person with Down syndrome, mostly unattractive, have always been present in our literature. Benjamin Compson, Faulkner's shuffling idiot narrator in *The Sound and the Fury*, is based on a character with Down syndrome, and it's not hard to find similar examples — the sad-eyed Mongol in *Take Me to Paris Johnny* and the 'retarded Mongol brother' with the mismatched ears in *The Jane Austen Book Club* are just two. As every parent of a child with Down syndrome is told though, 'Of course, things are so much better now!' *The Memory Keeper's Daughter*, an enormously popular recent novel which focuses on a baby with Down syndrome relinquished at birth, is light years away from *Darcy's Utopia*.

Today, for those who look, there are many positive depictions of people with Down syndrome in circulation in Australia: television programs such as the memorable SBS series *House Gang*, for example, which featured a group house occupied by people with intellectual disabilities, and the US TV series *Life Goes On*, starring Chris Burke. Pascal Duquenne was the Cannes award-winning star of the 1996 Belgian movie *The Eighth Day* and in 2009, the Spanish actor with Down syndrome Pablo Pineda was awarded the prize for best actor for his role in the movie *Me Too*. In the United Kingdom the fabulous 'docu-soap' *The Specials*, filmed in a household of young people with disabilities including Down syndrome, is great viewing.

Like the concurrent process of 'mainstreaming' Indigenous and ethnic Australians in the media, people with disabilities such as Down syndrome are starting to become more visible as pleasant, even popular incidental characters in mainstream productions. The former Australian television series *GP* featured the engaging Tracie Sammut as a regular cast member; *EastEnders* now features a baby with Down syndrome, and Australian actor Danny Alsabbagh appeared as Toby in the recent ABC TV series *Summer Heights High*. People with Down syndrome have appeared in Target catalogues and in advertising for ABC TV. In 2009 the short film *Be My Brother*, about a young man with Down syndrome, carried off first prize at Tropfest in Sydney for director Genevieve Clay while the lead actor Gerard O'Dwyer (who has Down syndrome) won the award for best actor.

Clearly, disability is now viewed more positively than was the case just a generation ago. Yet the birth of a child with Down syndrome still causes immense grief and untold anxiety for the family involved. The US term 'retard' has replaced the term 'spaz' (a favourite when I was a teenager) as a contemporary term of abuse among younger people. In Australia in May 2008, the Seven network's television series *All Saints* featured a young couple — brother and sister — who were expecting a child, and who were told that because the relationship was incestuous, the baby would have Down syndrome. The continuing currency of these sorts of images and this type of extraordinary misinformation makes a family's immediate response to the news that their child has Down syndrome and an intellectual disability at best ambivalent.

Tied up with the anticipated arrival of a baby is the expectation that the child will bring joy and happiness to the parents. Implicitly, a child is often seen as an extension of one's family, a link with both past and future. Most parents, particularly during their first experience of parenthood, marvel at the perfection which is their new child, and there can be few who have not harboured secret dreams and expectations. If we don't necessarily yearn to parent prime ministers and brain surgeons, most of us hope at the very least for the health, happiness and, ultimately, future independence of our offspring. At first glance, the birth of a child with Down syndrome seems to dash each one of these aspirations.

In not so distant days, the diagnosis of Down syndrome was so awful that parents were told to abandon all hope for a normal life with or for that child and to pass their Mongol baby straight into the hands of an institution. The legacy of that process of systematic abandonment is still with us today. If Down syndrome is a condition we can test for and screen against; if carrying a baby with Down syndrome is unquestioned grounds for termination; if bringing up a child with Down syndrome was once considered so dreadful a fate that people 'put their child away' instead, then the message is very clear: such a child is something to guard against, not to welcome. What kind of future are we opting for if we accept this child into our home? It is this question in all its starkness which parents have to confront when they learn the news about their newborn child.

Almost all parents of a child with Down syndrome remember the birth and the subsequent diagnosis in extraordinary detail as one of life's most profound watershed moments. The memories are fixed, a mental video to be painfully replayed over and over again. First-time parent Britt Canning's son Jack was born in 1995 at a hospital in Perth's northern suburbs. Britt described receiving the news as 'a huge shock, probably the biggest shock I have ever had and maybe ever will have, touch wood.' She and her husband were left 'quite shattered, absolutely devastated.'

> Looking back now, it was kind of bitter-sweet, it was both the worst and the best day of my life. It was quite a textbook labour, nine hours and no problems; he was born normally, naturally. He was a big baby too, a good size. I just remember once he was born I was in heaven, I was totally ecstatic. He breastfed straight away, he got an eight and then a nine in the APGAR[16] test and he was obviously just thriving.

> At about nine o'clock, the paediatrician came in to see me. Jack was lying in a bassinet at the time, I was sitting on the side of the bed feeling great, feeling really good. The paediatrician picked Jack up and put him in my arms and then he said to me, 'Have you heard of a condition called Down syndrome?' and my world just fell apart, just like that, those words. We were just absolutely shocked. I was holding Jack but I felt numb, completely numb. Now I wonder if it was such a good idea to give him to me, it is amazing I didn't actually drop him on the spot.

Luke Middleton recalled similar sensations.

> I felt absolutely devastated. I remember going outside and sitting on a park bench at the front of the hospital and everything seemed black and dark. I remember thinking that this was a terrible tragedy, a really terrible tragedy, and that all my wishes had collapsed.

Shock, horror and outrage went hand in hand with feelings of numbness, denial and total disbelief, all underpinned by a profound sense of sorrow and loss: loss of the perfect child whose arrival had been so eagerly anticipated, and loss of a way of life that had been taken for granted. Talking of this moment, people spoke in terms of their world falling apart, the end of life as they knew it; of devastation, anguish and mourning. For many parents, the death of their newborn child could scarcely have been worse and, initially at least, one of the most common sensations was of bereavement.

Recognition by medical staff that a child has Down syndrome is usually almost immediate. The condition is marked by a cluster of certain features which together constitute the 'syndrome' identified by John Langdon Down in 1866. While most of the public can identify people with Down syndrome from the distinctive appearance of their eyes, not all people with Down syndrome share this feature to the same extent, and this is not the feature medical staff rely on for immediate identification. The classical features (or 'stigmata', the technical term) of Down syndrome are visible in the face, neck, feet and hands. The eyes may appear to tilt upwards and be almond-shaped, a fact which led to earlier naming of the syndrome as 'Mongolism', as this feature was viewed as typically 'Asiatic'. The irises, particularly in fair children, sometimes exhibit rather attractive light flecks called 'Brushfield spots'. In some children, the tongue can protrude a little, and the mouth and its cavity may be smaller than normal. Ears too are sometimes smaller and the tips slightly folded over. A child's face sometimes appears flatter, especially the bridge of the nose, and the head smaller. Some children with Down syndrome have a characteristic transverse palmar or 'simian' crease, a single line crossing the palm of the hand instead of two; others have an inward curved little finger. Sometimes a wide gap exists between the first and the second toe.[17]

Low muscle tone (hypotonia), which gives the newborn child with Down syndrome its characteristic floppiness, is generally one of the first signs alerting medical staff to the presence of the condition. Some of the 'stigmata', particularly the smaller facial features, have medical implications, but hypotonia is the most significant as it can impact on the rate of a child's physical development. For that reason, while Down syndrome is typically thought of as an intellectual disability, it is also accompanied by delayed physical development in macro areas such as standing and walking, and in micro skills such as grasping and picking up objects. Low facial and oral muscle tone, often responsible for a protruding tongue, can also compromise or delay the child's ability to take solid food or to speak clearly.

As most recent books on Down syndrome are quick to point out, there is no correlation between the number of characteristic physical features a person with Down syndrome has, and their intellectual capacity. While that may be comforting later on, the knowledge that one has a child who can be identified as 'different' from the moment of birth is not.

Once the visible physical features have been noted, a medical practitioner will usually inform the family that Down syndrome is suspected, and that this can only be confirmed by a blood test. Usually the child and both parents are tested, to confirm the clinical diagnosis and to determine whether, as occurs in a very few cases, either of the parents is a 'carrier'. But generally the blood test will not answer the pressing question — *why us?* Apart from the knowledge that the incidence of Down syndrome does increase with maternal age, there is still no explanation for its occurrence.

A blood test, or cytogenetics report, clarifies the type of Down syndrome which the child has. Ninety-five per cent of cases occur in the form of trisomy 21, in which every 21st chromosome forms in triplicate instead of the usual twin form. Trisomy 21 has no apparent genetic implications. It is not 'carried' or passed from one generation to the next, and to date there is no explanation for this aberrant chromosomal formation. We do know that it occurs naturally in all cultures, though the rate varies according to the age profile of child-bearing women. In Western Australia, Down syndrome occurs in about one in 445 pregnancies.[18]

Down syndrome also occurs in two other forms: mosaic and translocation. Mosaicism occurs when not all of the body's cells are trisomic: some cells are normal and some have a third 21st chromosome, distributed in a random or 'mosaic' fashion. This condition has been described as 'incomplete' or 'partial' Down syndrome, and occurs in about four per cent of the population with Down syndrome. The condition is the subject of some research and debate because the extent and impact of the disability may be less than for other forms of Down syndrome.[19] Swimmers with mosaic Down syndrome, for example, compete for records in a separate category from swimmers with trisomy 21 as their performances are not always comparable. Sometimes too the condition may take longer to be identified, as was the case with Graham King in Geraldton whose mosaic Down syndrome was not diagnosed until he was five years old.[20]

Translocation Down syndrome, the least common form of all, is a condition where the extra 21st chromosome is not attached to the twin 21st chromosomes, but to another chromosome. This seems to be of no additional significance for the child, whose development and appearance will be 'typical' of children with trisomy 21, but it can sometimes have implication for the parents, as this form of Down syndrome may occur where one of the parents themselves has some translocated genetic material.[21] This is not always the case however, as Trish Weston was well aware.

Will has translocation Down syndrome, and it caused us massive angst waiting for our chromosome tests, to see which one of us was a carrier (the paediatrician had said one of us 'must be'). Will was the first grandchild on both sides and the implications for our siblings and their future children also seemed to be in the balance. It turned out that neither of us was a carrier.

The few days between initial diagnosis and confirmation by blood test are often days of great anxiety and roller-coaster emotions. These days, doctors tend to communicate their belief that the child has Down syndrome soon after the clinical examination, although this may also vary according to hospital policy or the doctor's inclination. When Catherine Slater's daughter Karen was born in May 1979, the London hospital where she was born had a policy of delaying passing on the news.

> If there was anything wrong, they wouldn't tell you for five days, for fear the mother might reject the baby. So everyone knew, but no one was telling me. I had absolutely no idea. I noticed nothing different from my first daughter; all you knew in those days about Down's syndrome was photos of people with pudding-bowl haircuts.

When the news finally did come,

> It was terrible. We'd had all the congratulatory cards from our friends and our family and everything. I couldn't ring anyone to tell them. I just couldn't.[22]

More recently in Perth, one family was denied knowledge of the clinical diagnosis even though trisomy 21 had been mentioned in the hospital case notes. The family was already very familiar with the condition as it had three adopted members with Down syndrome.

The doctors hadn't told them what their suspicions were. They were simply saying, we need to do some tests and Robert had read the file and because of our family, as soon as he saw trisomy 21 he thought, hang on, I know what that is. It was probably a week before the doctors in the hospital were prepared to even suggest that this child might have Down syndrome. They were just playing the game, 'We have to wait till this blood test comes back.' (Helen Golding)

Certainly, once they have informed the parents, doctors generally play down any possibility that their initial diagnosis might prove incorrect. Our doctor, for example, pointed out that if our daughter didn't have Down syndrome, she clearly had something else 'wrong' with her. Nonetheless, parents invariably hope against hope that there has been a mistake. Yet it is generally the initial news of the possibility of Down syndrome rather than confirmation by blood test which is remembered most clearly and most shockingly as the moment when the world fell apart.

What is the best way to break such news? Most parents felt that they should have been informed as soon as there was any diagnosis made by medical staff. But often it was the way in which the news was conveyed as much as the timing which compounded the distress, as was the case after Karen Langley and Paolo da Silva's daughter was born.

The paediatrician arrived and examined Shannon and then said, 'There is a heart murmur, but I don't know how serious it is at this stage.' And then he said, 'But I have to tell you I have concerns about your baby. I think this may be a Downs baby.' We were on the hospital bed and I think the main midwife from the Birthing Centre was there as well, and probably the others were all hovering in the background. Paolo said something like, 'What are you saying? Does she, or doesn't she?' Because the way he'd put it suggested that she might have; and then he said something which confirmed it. At that point, Paolo burst into tears.

For Loretta Muller, bad as the news was, she believed it had been well handled.

Initially the nursing staff said that they had some concerns because Cameron was born a little bit blue, and so they were talking about that rather than anything else. They weren't saying anything. Although later the midwife came down and said she knew as soon as he was born. But I didn't notice — I didn't know anything about babies! And then the paediatrician wanted to talk to me and my husband and so they took us aside and explained what they thought. He had several signs that suggested he may have Down syndrome, and as for everything else, he was fine. I thought it was really well done. It was without any prejudice. I never got the 'I'm sorry to tell you' or any of that. It was just, 'Look, we think this child has Down syndrome.' That was fine. 'We'll do some tests and we'll see what happens.' I was very shocked but I just thought, 'Poor little bugger.' Really, I thought, we'll just wait and see what happens.

When William Mann went to the hospital to see his wife Muriel on the afternoon of their son's birth in 1967, he was ushered into a little nurse's pantry off the ward where their doctor and an attendant paediatrician informed him that the child had 'Mongolism' and then left William to explain this condition and its consequences to his wife. He hadn't even seen the baby. Even worse was the experience of Mavis Simpson in 1943, who did not receive the news until well after she had taken her son Trevor home.

When I went back to the doctor — after you come home from hospital, you go back after a short period — then the doctor told me. It was a lady doctor and she was a very nice person. But, of course, it was a shock to us.

The different spheres of responsibility of doctors and nurses also determine when the news is passed on. In quite a number of cases, parents had to wait till the appropriate medical staff were present. When Shannon was born in Canberra, her mother Karen had no idea of her disability until thirty-six hours or so after she was born.

She happened to be born in the early hours of Sunday morning, when there wasn't a paediatrician available, who was the only person authorised to tell us. So the midwives knew and the doctor who delivered her knew, but nobody could actually tell us, which at the time upset me enormously ...

Almost instantaneously, when Shannon was born, the midwife who had been there all through my labour and the birth sort of closed up and she just wasn't the person that she had been before. And she actually came to me a day later and apologised that she hadn't been able to handle it. She saw the baby had Down syndrome. She knew she wasn't allowed to say anything and she just couldn't relate to the whole situation. But it was strange, that I had noticed the difference in her and there was actually good reason for it.

As a former nurse Trish Weston was well aware of the difficulties faced by staff having to withhold information, particularly when it is evident the parents are actively concerned about the child's condition.

The nursing staff were particularly supportive once they knew that I knew. Before that though, they really were tiptoeing around the edges, unable to say anything and feeling very uncomfortable about it. I mean, you can just sense that happening all around you. I think it was actively discussed, I've gathered that everyone kind of knew, but things weren't really allowed to be said.

Everyone knew the news was bad, but what it actually meant beyond that was seldom clear. Most fears about the future were based on understandable ignorance and in retrospect, some parents were even able to scoff at their own and their family's responses. Pamela Franklin recalled with laughter how, immediately after she had received her daughter's diagnosis, her first thought was, 'How am I going to go shopping with this kid?'

I thought people would look at me and look at her and that sort of thing. I don't know why it was shopping, it is not as though I really love going shopping or anything, I don't know why I thought that but I did. And my mother-in-law thought, how was she going to tell the bowling ladies?

After his daughter was born in 1995, Nigel Lawson wrote of his grief 'at the thought that Domenica's life expectancy is not much more than half her elder sister's.'[23] The belief that people with Down syndrome still have a much shorter life expectancy than the rest of the population is incorrect, but these and other sorts of misapprehensions about their child's future all contribute to the despair which usually follows a diagnosis of Down syndrome. Most parents felt they had lost any chance of a normal life for themselves and their families. Later on, the feeling that life *could* remain normal — whatever 'normal' might mean in the context of welcoming any new baby into one's household — became a source of great comfort. Yet it was the apparent certainty that a life shared with a child with a disability would always be different that most disturbed Helen Golding when her first grandson was born. She herself had three adopted children with Down syndrome, but she described her feelings when her eldest son Robert (who did not have Down syndrome) had a child with Down syndrome in 1992, in terms of deep shock.

> I was very upset. I was distressed because I knew that it meant that their life was not what they had thought it was going to be. Not because he is disabled, that doesn't matter a damn. But because I knew that from that day onward their life was not going to be the road they had thought it was going to be.

None of these families had had any idea of the news awaiting them. Kathy Evans in *Tuesday's Child* talks of her horror pregnancy with her daughter Caoimhe, and notes, 'Later I discovered that mothers carrying babies with chromosomal abnormalities can be sick the entire length of the pregnancy.' But this doesn't correlate with the experience of any of the women I interviewed, many of whom recalled that the pregnancy with the child with Down syndrome had been 'their best,' a model. At least two, however, did recall a 'fey' moment during the pregnancy, perhaps amounting to little more than what many mothers experience awaiting the birth of a child, especially their first. Britt Canning had recorded the moment in her diary.

> Towards the end of my pregnancy with Jack, I wrote in my journal that this has been the perfect pregnancy, no sickness, feeling wonderful, feeling better than ever, I hope

I am not being set up for a fall. I read that a couple of months later and it just gave me goose bumps, and it is almost like I did have a little premonition, and I mentioned it in a couple more entries towards the end, 'I just hope this isn't setting me up.'

Karen Langley recalled a similar experience.

There's two things I remembered about the pregnancy afterwards in relation to the Down syndrome. When we had our scan, I said to the woman who did it, 'Oh, and there's no sign of Down syndrome or something like that?' almost like a joke. And I remember her shaking her head, but in a sort of thoughtful way, and not actually saying no, and it's haunted me ever since that maybe she saw something and didn't feel like saying it or wasn't able to say it or whatever. The other thing is, our family doctor — I must have talked to her about the possibility of various difficulties and I remember her clearly, she said, 'I would put money on the fact that this baby will be normal.' I went back and told her after Shannon was born that she had said that to me, and she sort of looked at the sky and said, 'Oh, did I?'

The birth of a child with a difference can have the effect of making one feel totally isolated, underlining the feeling that one has been specially singled out. This was particularly the case for younger women who had a baby with Down syndrome. The 'why me?' element was foremost in many women's thoughts in the early days after the birth and was often reinforced by comments from friends and family. Britt, in her mid twenties when her first son was born, was struck by people's assumption that she was somehow responsible for her son's condition.

I didn't feel guilty myself — I felt more that other people assumed my guilt. No, I absolved myself pretty early on, but a relative wrote to me actually saying that you must feel terribly guilty about it as well. And I remember thinking, 'Well, I don't actually.' And still to this day when I think about that man, I feel like writing back to him and saying, 'You know, it wasn't necessarily me.'

One of the coping strategies sometimes adopted by parents of children with disabilities such as Down syndrome, and exemplified in Dale Evans' 1953 book *Angel Unaware*, was to label their children as 'gifts from God' given only to special parents 'chosen' for their capacity to cope, but that attitude certainly seems less common these days. None of the parents I interviewed saw themselves or their children in this light.

I was angry and I suppose I was angry in a religious sense. I thought, 'How dare God do this to me, I have tried to do the right thing by Him.' But I got all that over with, out of the way and just got on with it. (Pamela Franklin)

The belief that children with Down syndrome are only born to older mothers remains widespread and indeed, some family and friends seem to think that if a woman had a child with Down syndrome then it was her own fault for not taking proper precautions. When Luke Middleton rang his sister with the news, her first response was, 'Didn't she have the test?' Given the prevalence of the view that maternal age was the cause, younger women felt particularly called upon to account for their child's disability. In the absence of years, they surely must have had some other hidden flaw. At the very least, they usually felt they had been particularly hard done by.

Then there was the older mother bit too — that was also hard for people to understand. They said, 'Why has this happened to you? It shouldn't have happened to you!' and I felt that too! But yes, that was one of my first reactions: why did this happen to *me*? Then I looked at the odds of it happening, and I thought, oh great! (Britt Canning)

Maternal age is certainly a factor, with women over thirty-five more likely than younger women to have a child with Down syndrome. However, most children with Down syndrome are born to younger women simply because so many more women below thirty-five have children and, until very recently, fewer had prenatal screening for conditions such as Down syndrome.

Most people want to know why this has happened to them, and in the absence of any clear-cut answers, many look at their own lifestyles and prenatal experience. Trish Weston had worked many years in a hospital.

Had I been exposed to too many X-rays when I was working in the emergency department and those sorts of things? I worked in theatre for quite a long time, and the gases there are known to cause birth defects. I mean, that had been ten years before anyway, but I guess I was just searching for a reason why this had happened. I felt somewhat resentful of other people I knew whose babies were just fine, despite the fact that they smoked and drank through pregnancy and I'd done all the right things. I guess I felt like there was no justice really!

Scientist William Mann actively sought explanations when his son Geoffrey was born in 1967.

The librarian at the biological sciences library got books for me, everything that she could find on Down syndrome and at that stage, it was still regarded as being a maternal cause. There was a lot of rubbish written about Down syndrome. The book which reported the French discoveries spoke of things in genetic terms, and I could understand that, so it made sense.[24] But the best book that I read at the time was Down's original book.[25] It was really very informative.

Whether or not it helps parents to be able to point a finger and say, 'That might have been the trigger,' there remains no explanation for Down syndrome.

Getting a straight diagnosis can be complicated by the child's ethnic origins. In cases where the family had an Asian or non–Anglo Celtic background, aspects to the child's appearance which might otherwise have alerted a doctor to consider the possibility of Down syndrome were sometimes overlooked, as Brenda Harvey discovered when her daughter Grace was born in 1992.

> I didn't know Grace had Down syndrome until five days after she was born. Looking at her, you couldn't tell. Because they have an Indian father, my girls have always had that Asian look to them. And then the worst part was the waiting, five days of waiting, and not really knowing what I was waiting for. And I asked our doctor what did he think, and he looked at Grace and said, 'Well, she has some of the features but not all of them, so it's possible that she is Down syndrome but probably not.' Anyway, on the fifth day we had the results and my doctor came and told me that she did have it and so even though it was half expected, it was still a shock.

Claudia Mansour, who was originally from Lebanon, had to wait a great deal longer for the truth when her daughter Theresa was born in 1976.

No one detected anything wrong with Theresa. She had the slant eyes and also she had the very sparse hair whereas my other two were born with a lot of hair. And the obstetrician said, 'You people of the Middle East have almond eyes, so Theresa will have almond eyes ... and she will probably be a blonde,' and I never thought of it any further ...

When she was about four and a half months old she had a bit of a rash. So I rang up my GP and he said, yes, he wanted to see Theresa; he had not seen her. And as soon as he checked her up, the expression on his face was very weird. And he sat me down and he said, 'I think Theresa should have a chromosome test.' And I said, 'What for, what is wrong with her?' Straight away it ignited my doubts, you know. She was a very placid baby, just placid. But when I picked her up, often I used to think, she is a bit floppy. The other thing I noticed was that she didn't lift her head like other kids. I had seen all these things, but I couldn't really put my finger on them because I was assured that she was fine. So when the doctor told me, he sat me down and said, 'Look, do you see the knuckles on her fingers and the short fingers and the slant eyes, the low bridge nose, especially the muscles in the tummy, the soft muscles, the protruding tummy? We'll do the chromosome test, but I think Theresa is a Down.' I was totally devastated ...

So we went for the chromosome test. But when I took her the specialist assured me that there was nothing wrong. He said, 'She has beautiful long fingers like you, and I don't think I'd worry about it.' But I said, 'I would like to have it done.' I think they were the longest days in my life waiting by the phone. Ten days later the secretary of the specialist rang me up and she said, 'I would like you and Mr Mansour to come down to the surgery.' And this is when I really knew there was something wrong.

Notably, while the doctor who believed Theresa had Down syndrome saw her fingers as short and stubby, the specialist who was convinced she did not described the baby's fingers as long and slender like her mother's. As most parents of children with disabilities learn very quickly, preconceptions and prejudices about the condition are hugely important in determining how people with Down syndrome are viewed. Brenda Harvey recognised this while waiting for her daughter's diagnosis.

That five days I spent just sort of staring at her, and her face would just change before my eyes. One minute she'd look like my eldest daughter, the next minute she was like the other daughter and then the next minute she had a very Mongoloid look to her and looked like, very much like a Down syndrome baby. And then at other times she didn't look like that at all. So I don't think her face was really changing, I think it's just how we perceive it. And I mean that even happens now. I look at her and she's just so exquisite — exquisitely beautiful — and other times I see her and I think, oh yes, she does look a little bit Down syndrome, you know, but most of the time I don't see it at all.

The question of ethnicity was also raised when Britt Canning was given the news about Jack.

Before he even mentioned Down syndrome, the doctor asked if there was any Asian blood in our background. And I said, 'No. Mediterranean, but not Asian,' and that was when he brought up that they had noticed different things about

Jack, something to do with the shape of his head, a crease on the bottom of his feet. He said that they would have to do some blood tests to verify it but he believed there was a strong possibility that Jack had Down syndrome.

When Sandra Rossi was born in 1975 in the Kimberley in far northern Western Australia, doctors there took a number of weeks before they acknowledged that she had Down syndrome, again probably because of Sandra's ethnicity. Her mother Janet, though, 'knew something was wrong'.

Even though I was an enrolled nurse and I've nursed children, I've never really had much to do with the Downs, but I knew enough to know there was something wrong. They didn't tell me anything straight away. I was in hospital for maybe two weeks because she had a poor sucking reflex and she was floppy and all the typical sort of traits. I kept asking questions but they wouldn't answer me. They said it was fine, yet they wouldn't release me from hospital and then they started asking all sorts of questions about my background and my origin. My background is Chinese Aboriginal and my husband is Italian. Sandra had the stocky hands and fingers and features and the squinty eyes and stuff like that. They didn't know whether that was from the background, my genetic background, or from the Downs. A lot of the mixed Asian blood children do have the Mongoloid blotching on their backs. They found that confusing too. Yes, so in the end I was kept in suspense and I got a little bit depressed.

Parents — mothers more often than fathers and, more particularly, women who had already had a child or else had a nursing background — were often quicker than the medical staff to voice a concern that there was something a little different about their child. Pamela Franklin was already the mother of three when her daughter Catherine was born in 1984.

> The birth was fine but I knew immediately that there was something wrong with her. She just looked different to me and she didn't suckle. So, it was really funny, the doctor came over, he looked at her hand but one of her hands has got the very prominent simian crease (which I didn't know anything about then anyway), but the crease is a bit less marked on her other hand and he must have picked up that hand and looked at that. He picked up the nape of her neck and let her head drop back, and she seemed to be quite strong, he thought. He said, 'Look, she is fine,' and off he went ...

> But I said, 'I think she's got Down syndrome.' Anyway they took her away and I think they knew straight away, not that they told me. So they came back and said, 'We'll get a paediatrician in to have a look and that will set your mind at rest' — knowing, I think, full well that it wouldn't. So the paediatrician came in and confirmed it for me. But I had been hoping against hope that I was wrong. So it was still a shock and my husband was absolutely devastated, he was beside himself. This was only two hours after the birth. The paediatrician said you can have the test, but she had two toes that stuck out, she had the palmar creases, she had the speckled eyes and all those sorts of things. Of course, I hadn't known to pick up all those things; all it was to me was that she looked different.

Trish Weston had similar concerns almost immediately after her firstborn son Will arrived. One can only wonder at the logic of ignoring the well-founded and openly expressed fears of an anxious parent.

There was a very short period of time after he was born, I was still in the delivery suite, where I didn't realise, but once I actually held him and looked at him and he didn't want to suckle straight away, I thought, 'Hmm, yes, something here.' I just knew there was something wrong. I have a nursing background and I've seen babies born and I know what babies ought to look like at birth.

So, I had the first inklings, but I decided not to listen! And then the paediatrician said we're going to run some tests, but unfortunately, we had a paediatrician who was very evasive and told us these were quite normal. Again, because of my training, I knew that this wasn't a normal sort of a thing at all ...

Michael was so excited and elated, he just said, 'Oh no, I'm sure you're wrong,' but I said, 'I know there's something wrong.' I had those feelings of elation too — I still did — but there was this kind of thing hovering around in the background that was a bit of a worry. But no one was telling us what the problem was.

In the end it was the obstetrician who delivered Will who I spoke to about it. I said, 'Look, I'm fine, don't worry about me, but I'm worried about the baby.' And he said, 'What do you think is wrong?' And I had to say, 'I think he has Down syndrome.'

I still get *so angry* that the obstetrician made me actually put into words what I was really worried about. I think it would have been far kinder for them to have taken that opportunity, when I said I think there's something wrong, to have said, 'Well yes, we are worried,' and so forth, but they made me ... they made me say it. And then he said, 'Yes, that is what we're concerned about and that is what we are testing for.' And I guess that's when my world fell apart. I am still very bitter about that experience.

Iris Fisher, also a former nurse, was present when her granddaughter Trudy was born in 1979 and was quick to recognise her condition. Her fifteen year old daughter Sally, who was at that stage in the care of the Department of Community Welfare as a runaway, had been living a hard life and Iris had some concerns about the child's health even before it was born.

When Trudy was born, I was present at the birth. I had anticipated that Sally would have a sick baby and a poorly nourished one because her breakfast would be a cigarette. And she was drinking, so you already had the factors of a mother who smoked and drank. And I knew that we could have on our hands a very sick baby. At birth, it was touch and go whether Trudy would survive, but she did. It was during that night that I said to my husband, 'I think she's a Down syndrome.' The next day, we went to the hospital and to start off they wouldn't let us see the baby. I said that I'd been present at the birth and my husband actually turned to the sister and said, 'My wife thinks that Trudy could be a Down syndrome child,' and they were very surprised because it wasn't really all that obvious at that point. They had suspected but they were surprised that I had picked it up. This possibly was due to the few I'd seen born during my year of midwifery. Otherwise, I'd had no contact with Down syndrome people at all.

Letting other people know about the new baby's condition was sometimes a big hurdle for new parents who needed their family's support and honesty but were wary of their reactions.

Faced with their own disbelief, shock and uncertainty, the prospect of supporting an extended grieving family was more than some wanted to handle. Explaining to an older generation, with an even greater legacy of negativity towards disabilities such as Down syndrome, when the parents themselves still knew very little about the condition, was at best challenging, but most grandparents seemed to handle the news with dignity.

> They didn't really show us how deeply they were hurt and I think that's something that we're grateful for, that they did provide support in that way that we didn't have to go out and support them as some people do. But what was a bit difficult was, I think, perhaps not insinuations, but just comments like, 'Oh well, you know, we haven't had anything like that in our side of the family.' And they obviously don't realise the implications of what they are saying! But there was a little bit of that. (Trish Weston)

Quite often, well-meaning friends and family will say of a baby with Down syndrome, 'Oh, he looks fine,' or, 'She doesn't look like she has Down syndrome so she is bound to be all right!' not realising that the so-called 'typical' features, the distinctive eyes, are not the only physical characteristic indicating the presence of Down syndrome. For distraught new parents like Mary Tanaka, whose family has an Asian Aboriginal background, this can appear as denial.

> My husband rang up my parents and his parents and it was all, 'Oh no, it's all right!' and that sort of thing. And I had my aunt and uncle, and my in-laws and my parents all there at the hospital, and they were all saying, 'Oh no, they've made a mistake. He's perfect. He looks wonderful. He looks all right!' And the doctor, not five minutes before, told me he

definitely had Down syndrome! So that was the hardest thing. That really upset me. They weren't accepting it and I don't know if they were trying to make me feel better, but they didn't. It made me worse. It's the denial, I think. It would have been easier if they had just accepted it, but they kept saying, 'Oh, no, he's perfect!' and, 'Oh no, the doctors have made a mistake. No, he just looks Japanese!' So I think that was the hardest. But I think on the other hand, if they had broken down and cried, that would have made me feel bad too, so I don't know where the balance is.

Certainly, parents found their extended family's response to the news influenced how they themselves coped.

The best thing that happened to me was that I immediately rang my mum. I said, 'Oh, they think the baby has got Down syndrome,' and she said, 'Gee, that is a bit of bad luck.' And it was just like that. And I thought, 'Oh,' and then I was fine and it was just, what can you do? If he has, he has; if he hasn't, then he hasn't. That was really levelling for me and it put it all in perspective and it was just fine. It wasn't a drama and that was really good. I think Andrew's family found it harder and they were hoping that the tests would come back and that everything would be all right and I think that was kind of hard. (Loretta Muller)

Luke Middleton also appreciated his family's support.

My sister rang back to tell me she'd been to see a friend of hers who had a seventeen year old daughter with Down syndrome, who she said was just finishing high school. This was something of a revelation to me. It really tore me out of black despair. This friend of hers had told her about all that could be done now with early intervention and I began to feel very differently after that conversation. My brother and his wife came with bottles of baby champagne and toasted the baby, and neither of them was the slightest bit upset about the baby. So everybody was very supportive.

The friends of English racing car driver Damon Hill made a similar gesture of acceptance, insisting in the face of the family's initial reluctance that the baby be welcomed with champagne when Hill's son was born in the United Kingdom.[26] The significance of celebrating the baby's arrival was also important for Britt Canning.

In the midst of all of this I felt terribly guilty that we weren't celebrating Jack being born. You know, this child had been born into the world and everyone was grieving and upset and sad and so we kind of pulled ourselves together and Peter said, 'Well come on, let's pour the champagne, let's smoke the cigars and welcome this little baby.' So Mum and I drank champagne and I cried a little bit more.

Equally, friends and relatives took their behavioural cues from the parents.

I know afterwards people said that they found it much easier to accept his disability because I wasn't stressed out about it. They found that was easier for them because I had accepted it and so they felt they could as well. (Loretta Muller)

In Loretta's case, breaking the news had been handled well, and she had had the benefit of a supportive mother. Certainly, the capacity of new parents to be at least outwardly accepting of the diagnosis was often the result of how the news was conveyed in the first place — as a disaster or a fact of life —

and of how others responded to the news. For some parents though, no gesture of support could console them.

> My hospital room became like a funeral parlour, I had just so many flowers come in, I think people didn't know what to say, so they thought we'll just send flowers. They weren't sending me flowers out of joy; they were sending me flowers out of sympathy. (Heather Burton)

In some cases, cultural, religious and ethnic differences had an enormous impact on a family's ability to understand or accept their child's disability. Sunil Ravi came to terms with his child's disability by adopting a perspective on her condition which was at odds with his cultural inclinations but he knew that the medical approach he consciously embraced would not be accepted among the people he had grown up with in India. Although his daughter is now in her teens and has visited India three times with her family, Sunil's Indian relatives still haven't been told she has Down syndrome. He felt his parents and family would react negatively if they heard about his daughter's disability.

> When my brother came out with, 'Why is she like that, why is she very quiet?' I said, 'She's only shy.' I don't want to tell them ...

> I come from a different background, different culture, different customs, different beliefs. I'm a Christian, and I grew up in a community of Muslims, Hindus, other people. But anyway, all these people have got one thing in common. If something's wrong with your child, my child, his child, her child, it's God's curse on you. I'm not arguing the Australian perspective, I'm not arguing what's wrong or right, but arguing my point of view from my Indian background.

We believe many things, you know, but if something happens to someone, the first thing is everyone gets together, has a gossip, you know, the local gossip: 'Oh, he has done something before. Now he has to have a punishment' ...

My family would, I don't know, be with my friends or some other relatives, or cousins or somebody who doesn't like me, or who I don't like, they would have this kind of talk: 'Oh he must have done something in his past life,' or 'God is giving him a good punishment. Let him live with it for the rest of his life,' watching this girl grow up mentally handicapped. It's all part of the community. It's very hard to explain to you, unless you come and live there with me for twenty years.

Naturally, Sunil's cultural background determined his own response when his daughter Amber was born.

My first reaction was, I couldn't work it out. I thought, 'Oh, what big mistake have I made in the thirty years since I was born?' But I didn't make any major, major mistake like people in the world do, you know? It took me one year reading the books: 'Oh she's got an extra chromosome.' It happens once in a thousand, one in eight hundred, by accident. So I got into the reason, the medical thing, and it made more sense. So I know she's got Down syndrome, there's no doubt about that. But everything is changed now, I don't feel like that now.

The reaction of the baby's siblings was another critical factor in determining how parents came to terms with their new child. While parents approached breaking the news to their other, especially older, children with trepidation, what most discovered was a total lack of concern about issues such as disability. By the time Claudia Mansour knew of her daughter's diagnosis, baby Theresa was almost five months old, which made telling her other daughter and son that much more difficult and compounded her own distress about Theresa.

> How to break it to my children? I'd cry all day and when they came home my daughter would say, 'Mum, what is wrong?' I started to postpone it and postpone it. Then I went and saw my priest and he said, 'Well you just tell them the truth, when you feel ready.' One day I decided, okay, today I'm going to tell Anne. I said to her, 'Well, Theresa is going to be retarded, if you like; she won't be able; she's got Down syndrome. We don't know how bad she is going to be.' She said, 'Is that all, Mum? Is that what you were crying about? So what if Theresa is not as bright as we are to be? Do we stop loving her? Do you love your children just because they are beautiful and because they are intelligent?' It took me aback. I never thought of it that way and I thought, 'Gee, you really can learn from your kids.'

Children too young to understand about disability could also bring an entirely different dimension to responses to the new baby: normality.

> I remember saying to Ruth, who was three years old and had been waiting for this birth for such a long time, 'Look it's your new baby sister!' and feeling like I wanted to burst into tears. Ruth, of course, was completely amazed and delighted and rapt at this new little creature. And I think she was the only one who was utterly and completely un-ambivalent about this little baby. Ruth really helped because for her there was no other agenda, it was just, 'Here she is at last, my gorgeous baby sister,' and that really helped us enormously. (Jude Lawrence)

While family support can help parents accept a child's disability more quickly, when Mavis Simpson's son Trevor was born in 1943 some of her relatives were brutally frank, their attitudes in line with prevailing views of Down syndrome.

One of my uncles, who married later in life, had three children too, two girls and then a boy with Down syndrome, but that boy baby didn't live. And the mother of that baby said to me, when Trevor was born, 'Oh you should pray that he won't live; you know, that God will take him.' Which was an idea I couldn't fancy at all!

People were sympathetic, you know. They thought we'd had a very great misfortune and they must be very nice to us and so forth, and nobody was *rejecting* of him, but, you know, there weren't very many positive things you could say then, because there was so little available.

Thirty-five years later, when their granddaughter Trudy was born, Iris Fisher and her husband Des had much the same experience. 'Our expectations were very low. In fact, we were just sort of told, well, you know, virtually they were cabbages. Very little could be done.'

There is an idea that all people with Down syndrome look alike, but this generally stems from stereotypical social characteristics such as clothing, as much as chromosomes. The image, often associated with institutions, of shuffling people with Down syndrome with pudding-basin haircuts and worn-out ill-fitting clothes was one which struck many new parents forcefully — until they realised that in fact the way their kids dressed was entirely up to the parents! Parents saw themselves stereotyped too. Pamela Franklin feared that she would be forced into the mould of 'parent of disabled child'.

I always had that vision of those kids with baggy pants and shoes and socks and the bowl-cut hair and everything and I always used to look at people like that, and feel sorry for the mother, and it was always an older mother. *Those* were the things I remembered seeing and I didn't want to be the same as that.

Five years after the birth of her son, Mary Tanaka still pondered the child she had thought she was going to have. 'I've always wondered what he would look like. And I always thought that he would look like his brother more.' For her, the physical signs of Lucas's disability seemed to overshadow family characteristics. In spite of any 'typical' features however, people with Down syndrome generally carry clear family traits. Yet the stereotype that they resemble each other more than they do members of their own family is sometimes thoughtlessly fostered by doctors and health professionals.

The doctor said something which really hurt and which was, I know now, completely wrong. He said intellectually they vary tremendously, which was good, but he said in terms of appearance they all look pretty much the same. So suddenly all these images that I had in my head were confirmed, that this is how Jack would look. When he was a little baby I wasn't thinking of his intellect anyway and to be honest, the appearance side of it was what frightened me and upset me the most, because I suddenly felt as if he had been snatched away from us and put in a different group altogether. He wasn't a part of our family. I felt he wouldn't look like us, he wouldn't take after us in any way. He would be part of this separate group and the doctor I think quite unknowingly drove a bit of a wedge between us and Jack at that point. (Britt Canning)

Adapting to a new reality takes time for the parents of any child with a disability, especially after a period of desperate flirtation with denial. There may be some comfort though in the ruthless certainty of the verdict of Down syndrome. Parents of a child with a disability such as autism or a non-specific intellectual delay can live on a knife edge for years before confirmation of long-held fears. Though it seems to fall like a guillotine on the future, learning that one's child has Down syndrome may in fact be easier to live with than the inexorable paring away of hope which accompanies other less clearly identifiable developmental disabilities. That may be no consolation to the parents of a newborn, but the creep towards emotional acceptance, once begun, is generally a journey along a one-way street.

What most parents feared initially was that living with Down syndrome was a life sentence with hard labour.

> I had to give a speech to Rotary club, and I remember saying that they say when you die, your life flashes before you. I suppose I had the reverse, I had this vision of this life ahead of me that was going to be. I would be tied down forever with this person. I did think that and I was angry about that. I suppose I thought I was going to have a better life than that. (Pamela Franklin)

Realising that this 'life sentence' view was mistaken did a huge amount to help some people get back on track. Things as simple and normal as breastfeeding the baby were important. Some mothers were actively discouraged from trying, even told by medical staff (usually doctors) that babies with Down syndrome 'didn't breastfeed.' But for those who tried, like Loretta Muller, the experience was usually a positive one and contributed a great deal to the feeling of normality — that this was after all, just a newborn baby.

I remember being really disappointed because they gave him his first feed and that was a bottle feed. But no one told me I couldn't breastfeed him. So I just did and they were, 'Oh wow.' Then a week later when we had it all under control they said, 'This is very unusual.' So that was really nice.

Breastfeeding was also a catalyst in helping some mothers bond with the child.

I didn't really want to have anything to do with her, initially. The special nurse came in and asked me if I was going to feed her and I said no, not unless I had to. And so she took her away again, and then this other nurse came in the next morning and said, 'How are you going to feed her, are you going to breastfeed her or is she going to be bottle fed?' I said I didn't really give a so and so. So she immediately whipped her out of the bassinet and threw her on my breast and she helped her on and made sure that she did it. And I suppose that was really the beginning of the end. That was the best thing anyone ever did for me really. From then on I wasn't too bad at all. (Pamela Franklin)

Jude Lawrence also described how life began to assume more normal proportions even before she left hospital, because she was blessed with supportive friends and colleagues.

When Laura was born I started thinking, I'll never be able to go back to work, I'll have to stay home and look after this kid for the rest of my life; all this sort of bizarre stuff you think. But one person who came to see us almost immediately was the director of the day care centre that our elder daughter Ruth went to. We had assumed that Laura would go to day care when she was six months old or something. Then when she was born we thought, do kids with Down syndrome go to day care? We'd certainly never seen a child with Down syndrome at day care. Sylvia came to see us and said, 'Look I've worked in England with children with Down syndrome and there'll always be a place for your daughter in my centre.' And it started to seem almost immediately that life *would* go on, and the things I'd been intending to do, like eventually go back to work and use day care, that would all be possible too.

I was told a story second hand of a woman who, whenever she sees her grandson, shakes her head sadly and says, 'If only she had had the test!' This story may well say more about the grandmother than the child, but it underlines that acceptance — of the new direction life has taken and of one's new baby — may not be immediate, and it is certainly not universal. Heather Burton was one mother who battled for years. As part of the process of moving on after her daughter's birth in 1994, Heather approached the Butterfly Garden at the cemetery, where infants or stillborn babies are memorialised, with a view to placing a stone to commemorate the child who had *not* been born but whom she was still deeply mourning.

> You're desperate for this horrible sense of grief to disappear. And I think ... when you're wishing your child would die, it's not actually wishing your child would die, it's wishing that the grief would die ...

> So I rang up the cemetery and I've forgotten how I worded it, but I said, 'Well it wasn't a real child but it was real to me.' Anyway she talked it out with me and said, 'Look I'm terribly sorry, but it has to be a real child, so we can't offer you a space.'

Heather wisely sought counselling, and when she asked one

of her counsellors whether things would ever improve for her, he gave a qualified 'yes'.

He said, 'I do have a group of mothers who live their grief and they wallow in it and they socialise with other women who are in it and that's how they live.' I just thought well, I don't want to be there, I want to be able to get rid of this grief. I think for the most part I am now in that place where the grief is less intense and when it comes it might only last a day, or half a day — sometimes longer depending on the issue, if something's cropped up, or there's stress in the family at the time. But I can manage it a lot better because I'm a lot happier.

Other parents too, like Heather, frankly admitted that in their earliest darkest days, they had thought it might be easier if the child simply didn't survive, an emotion which was couched in terms both of what they thought best for the child and what they thought best for themselves and for their families: whether they were prepared or able to cope with what they thought the future held. In no case was the thought acknowledged as more than fleeting. However, with up to one-third of babies with Down syndrome being born with some degree of heart defect, acceptance for some families was undoubtedly complicated by the prospect of life-threatening heart surgery. Karen Langley spoke frankly and emotionally of the implications of this for her and husband Paolo da Silva.

It's hard to even say it now but I think we were sort of comforted by the fact that she'd got to have this major heart surgery and she might not survive. We went through those first few months as I would imagine anyone does who has a child that may not survive, not really ... or at least, *pretending* that we weren't *that* attached maybe. It wasn't like we were in some sort of rejection thing, I mean we were definitely there as full-on parents ... I just think there was just something *very different* on that morning after the surgery, running up to the intensive care unit when they called. They called us very early saying she might not survive and we ran all the way from the hostel place where we were staying at the back of the hospital to the ward, and I remember trying to talk in between running and saying that I realised I didn't care a shit about the Down syndrome, this baby had to survive. It had suddenly dawned on me that it was *really really* important. So, although I think we'd bonded with her before that, I think that was the first time that I really admitted to myself that yes, I did want this baby. I didn't care if she had Down syndrome.

For other parents, the fear that they could never love this child with a difference as much as they loved their others was a source of great anguish. As Richard Gregson poignantly explained, the belief that a child with Down syndrome would always be a responsibility to be borne, rather than a child to be loved, undermined his earliest thoughts about his son.

There was no question that we wouldn't take him in, and that we weren't the people for good or bad reasons that were responsible for his welfare. I mean, we gave birth and as far as I am concerned it is our responsibility. That didn't make it any easier to know whether we could deal with it. We were just taking one day at a time at that stage. We had no doubt that we *had* to deal with it. I guess there was this big void, this big doubt as to what extent we could feel the same way towards Jordan as we felt towards our daughter Miranda and to what extent we would feel that he was a member of our family ...

Acceptance didn't happen overnight. Jordan didn't smile until he was at least four months I think. I had a difficulty with it personally and I knew Beth was having difficulty. I will never forget how she said it. She was standing in the corridor, she had just picked up Jordan, she was taking him to his cot and she turned around and looked at me, and thought for a while whether she would say something, and then she said, 'Richard, I just can't feel anything for Jordan.' That is the first and only time that she has ever said anything remotely like that to me and I will never forget that. But I will also never forget the first time he smiled and I tell you, it took a few weeks but once you make that contact, you see the child behind the body and suddenly there is his soul, he is everything that Miranda ever was, you stop seeing the Downs and you just see your child.

Ultimately, for most parents, love for their child had a way of stealing up when they least expected it.

I can read back to my diary now — I was writing almost daily at that stage — but two weeks after he was born there was just this sudden transition. It had all been gloom and doom: 'I am so depressed,' and 'When is this going to end?' And then I woke up one morning, it was a beautiful day and I just couldn't wait to see Jack in the cot, I couldn't wait to see him and dress him up and I realised then that all these images I'd had of having a baby to do things with and play with and dress in lovely clothes — I thought that had been taken away from me, but it hadn't, and Jack *was* the baby I'd dreamed of having. It only took two weeks to reach that point, I had relapses of course along the way, but at that point there was no looking back, he was well and truly in our hearts to stay. (Britt Canning)

The birth of a baby with Down syndrome is too often experienced as a tragedy for the family concerned. But the real tragedy is the way in which the birth is presented to the family: as an inevitable source of deep pain and regret and the beginning of a long and bitter journey down a road *no one* would wish to take. This view can come from medical staff, friends and family, or simply from the parents' own understandings of the meaning of disability. Very quickly however, these outmoded ideas of the baby with Down syndrome as a burden to be borne begin to disappear, as families realise that this baby is, after all, just a baby, that the arrival of any new baby brings 'difference' to a household, and that life — theirs and their newborn child's — is very much worth living.

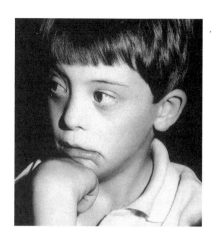

chapter 2
MAKING CHOICES

'If she had been born twenty years ago, you'd be going home through the front door and she'd be leaving out the back.'
(Nursing staff to Luke Middleton, father of newborn daughter with Down syndrome, 1992)

'We were just so inconvenient to them.'
(Emily Howard, who chose to proceed with a pregnancy after diagnosis of Down syndrome, 2008)

'I thought, what is another one, what difference does another one make?'
(Helen Golding, mother of two children with Down syndrome, on her decision to adopt a third)

Choices shape our lives. The previous chapter dealt with the situation where Down syndrome was 'thrust upon' unprepared and usually unwilling families, but there are many ways in which Down syndrome can be more actively 'chosen' or rejected. What we tend to regard as a personal choice — for example, the decision whether or not to go through with the pregnancy once a prenatal diagnosis is available — is always made within the context of social, cultural and community influences, few of which are straightforward or transparent. While personal circumstances influence decision-making, larger frames of reference determine the range of options available and how we respond to them.

There are more choices available today to families with a child with Down syndrome than there were for earlier generations. Formerly, when a child with a disability such as Down syndrome was born, parents would be encouraged to see that the best course of action was to put the child into state care, which meant institutionalisation. Parents were told to give it up and to go home: forget about it and have another one. This attitude is a less extreme version of the position espoused by bioethicist Peter Singer, who argued in *Practical Ethics* that just as the foetus is 'interchangeable or replaceable' should it die or be aborted before birth, so too is the newborn infant.[27] While Singer went further to argue that there is no ethical difference between the termination of a pregnancy with a disability or the termination of a newborn infant for the same reasons, our society to date has drawn the line at infanticide, though we are happy enough with abortions. In Western Australia until the 1960s, children with disabilities would typically have been placed at birth in institutions such as Claremont Hospital for the Insane, or later into Pyrton Training Centre, where they might spend their whole lives. Such children, if not entirely forgotten, sometimes became strangers to their families. When Kew Cottages for people with intellectual disabilities burned down in Melbourne in

1996, there were families in the community who had no idea they had close relatives living there.[28] Yet there were other parents who had never been able to do as they had been advised and simply move on and forget. As Corinne Manning shows in her book on Kew Cottages, the road to the institution was all too often 'a river of tears.'[29] Children, 'even' those with disabilities, are not always as easily replaced as Singer might suggest.

Mavis Simpson's son Trevor was lucky. Born in 1943, his family rejected the paediatrician's suggestion that institutionalisation was the best option.

> We saw the usual child specialist that people were referred to, but he didn't have anything much to tell us at all. And I asked him, you know, if there was any literature I could read or anything like that. He didn't think that was a good idea at all! He felt the right thing to do was to 'put him away,' as they said in those days. But, you know, that wasn't what we wanted, and so we didn't see him again. And we just kept in touch with our family doctor.

Geoffrey Mann was born in 1967. This was a time when in Western Australia at least, under the guidance of psychologist Guy Hamilton (appointed in 1964 to the position of super-intendent of the Mental Deficiency Division of the state's Mental Health Services), attitudes to institutionalisation were gradually changing.[30] Hamilton was in the Australian van-guard of moves to keep children with less severe disabilities such as Down syndrome at home with their families and his attitude to disability had wide-reaching implications for individual families and for people with disability more generally. The Mann family met with Hamilton soon after Geoffrey's birth and found they shared his views on keeping children with disabilities out of institutions. As William

Mann said of his wife, 'The maternal instinct came right to the fore. She was utterly and totally protective and wouldn't even consider relinquishing her babe.'

So Geoffrey was another child fortunate enough to grow up within his own family. Having made the decision to keep their children at home, Geoffrey's and Trevor's families both became mainstays of organisations like the Slow Learning Children's Group (SLCG), which were fundamental to facilitating changes on behalf of all families with disabilities such as Down syndrome.

Other Western Australian families also stared down the spectre of giving up their child to the state. Charlie King (born 1965) and Frank Flynn (born 1969) were both born into Aboriginal families in the Kimberley and their mothers were well aware from their own cultural backgrounds of the readiness with which state authorities had taken Aboriginal children from their families in the very recent past. Though they faced a fair degree of pressure, both were adamant that they would not give up their sons for any reason at all, not even for the temporary purposes of education or access to services down south. Aboriginal families had heard all that before.

Mum told this story about Charlie and she had to put on a bit of a fight and she went and spoke to one of her uncle-in-laws, her uncle, and he said to her, if you want your son, we'll go and support you all the way, so he supported her, him and his wife, which was my grandmother's sister, and she ended up with Charlie. (Marg King, Charlie's sister)

As a single parent with a large family, Frank Flynn's mother faced even greater pressures.

There was a double whammy of being part of the stolen generation, having children taken off you. So Mum was very strict about invasion of privacy by the Welfare, or by the social workers and that sort of stuff. It was like, you won't get my child off me; I am capable of looking after my child no matter what, even with this problem. But from the Welfare Department, it was just constant that you should put your child up for adoption, farm him off to someone else, or whatever. That was always there, yes, so that was a fear. (Denise Flynn, Frank's sister)

For other families too, the thought of institutionalisation was inconceivable. In 1964 the Benn family felt they were no longer able to deal with their four year old son who had an intellectual disability. They were utterly desperate about his future, but his mother would not countenance the thought of Irrabeena or an asylum. So his father shot him.[31] The tragedy became a cause célèbre across Australia, not as a reminder of the human rights of children with disabilities, but as a rallying point for arguing for better long-term accommodation facilities. Any notion of the child with a disability as a gift from God was completely replaced by the view of a child with a disability as a burden verging (for some) on the unbearable.

By the time most of the children in the families I interviewed were born, institutionalisation was no longer a possibility for children with disabilities. The expectation now was that children were best cared for in their own homes, and from the 1980s more state and private support was made available to help families do so. Even with that shift though, there were (and still are) alternatives available to a family that decides it doesn't want to take a child home.

Relinquishing a child, giving it up for adoption, was raised with one Australian family when Angus Grant was born in the United States in 1971. His father Bernard recalled the doctor saying, 'You don't have to have this child; you can send him off to a foster home.' But they didn't consider it.

> At first Angela had a huge shock and she, in a sense, rejected him, and didn't do breastfeeding. But we had decided before she and Angus left hospital that we would take Angus. Our pastor, who'd also visited us, suggested we keep him, and that was our natural inclination anyway, that we weren't going to reject him. It just seemed too cruel to say in effect, this child is not a person. We didn't feel pressured, I think it was just one of the options. I don't know that the doctor seriously would have pushed it, but he certainly made it clear that we wouldn't be thought badly of if we did that.

This father's thoughts encapsulate the two biggest issues for families contemplating relinquishing now, just decades since institutionalisation ceased to be the norm: is it cruel and unnatural, and what would other people think? Trish Weston's son was born in 1984 and she was shocked when she later realised that some families still gave up their children — despite the fact that she had earlier worked with children with disabilities in an institutional setting.

> That was so long ago and I always thought their families were poorer for having relinquished them. And when Will came along it wasn't an issue for us at all. Number one, we wanted him very much, we loved him very much right from the start no matter what. And we had no awareness that [relinquishing] was even an option. The opportunity was never presented. But I'm pleased that it wasn't because it would have given us something else to think about and to worry about and it might have coloured the way we felt about the whole situation. If you can give up the baby for adoption because of Down syndrome, what does this mean?

Is this going to be awful? A lot worse than we think it is? No. It was not until a social trainer said something about a family who had thought about relinquishing but didn't, that I realised ... I was quite stunned. I said, 'Do you mean that people actually still give up their babies because they have Down syndrome?' And she said, 'Oh yes, they do.' And that was just an absolute revelation to me. I have no judgement to make about anyone who does, but it was not something that we thought about doing.

Another mother hadn't realised that relinquishing was a possibility until her doctor mentioned it. This was in the early 1990s.

I remember being really distraught and my doctor saying to me at one stage, 'Well, people do give up their babies,' and I thought, 'Oh God, there's an open door!' But my husband said straight away, 'She's ours, we have to take her.' And he was right, and I knew it. Even asking the question in the first place, you know what the answer's going to be. And I think that was a turning point because from that moment I accepted that this was it, and life was going on, and she was part of our life. But perhaps to have confronted the possibility of letting her go so early and then to step back and say, 'No, that's not for us,' was good, I think.[32]

When the Goldings adopted Damian in 1983, the issue of adoption became a topic of extreme interest for the friends of Damian's new ten year old sister, and their questions captured common attitudes around the idea of giving up a child, with or without a disability: 'Did they give him up just because he had a disability?' 'Don't you think that is awful?' 'That was a horrible thing to do, they should've kept him.' Helen Golding however had a different perspective.

Everybody has to do what is right for them ... and to be able to say, 'I can't do this,' and give the child to someone who you think can do it better, I do think it is a very brave thing to do, knowing what it would be like to have a child and have to give it up. It wouldn't be an easy thing for anyone to do. People say, 'They take the easy road out.' Well, I don't think so, I don't think it is the easy way at all.

Certainly the reluctance of people to countenance relinquishing their child these days, even if it is not necessarily the child they had wanted, suggests that for whatever reason, it is still the harder road. The advent of deinstitutionalisation has shifted the ground considerably in terms of what is socially and personally acceptable. Families who would have contemplated a termination had they received a prenatal diagnosis of disability could not even begin to consider the prospect of relinquishing once the child was born; yet for a previous generation, letting go one's child with a disability had been the norm.

For those few families who do decide after a child is born that bringing up a child with a disability is not for them, the child can be fostered on a temporary basis, or it can be made available for adoption, which is irrevocable. Giving up a child for adoption involves an intensive process of consulting and counselling and there are safety nets for relinquishing families who might want to change their mind before the decision becomes absolute. As one adoptive parent explained however, even a temporary fostering situation can become long term and the absence of a firm decision to relinquish can impact adversely on the children involved.

There are some children whose parents are not prepared to raise them themselves but also who are not willing to put them up for adoption, and they spend their lives in foster homes, which is very sad because they really need for the natural parents to be prepared to make the decision one way or the other. Not to try and play it both ways and say, maybe in a couple of years I might be able to cope with you but I can't now, because if you can't cope with a baby [with Down syndrome] you won't cope with a toddler or a seventeen year old. (Helen Golding)

Even when parents do put their child up for adoption, the child can still remain in a foster home for a very extended period and as they age, their chances of finding an adoptive family diminish. Helen Golding adopted her third child with Down syndrome in 1989. Josie was two and a half when the family was approached by Community Services and asked if they could take her on.

She was actually released from hospital very early and she went straight to the foster home. Her parents had opted out of it a very long time ago and have never wanted any contact, any information. The foster parents that she was with were not prepared to have her long term. She could in fact have spent the rest of her life going from foster home to foster home. I guess it was more the uncertainty for her that sort of won me over in the end. I thought, what is another one, what difference does another one make?

When in 1983 she first began thinking about adopting a child with a disability, Helen already had two children, one of whom was adopted, and she had had some experience working with children with disabilities. Her children were growing up and she was looking for a different direction in her life.

I was reading the newspaper one morning and there was a huge notice, an advertisement really, from Community

Services. They had a list of about eight children with disabilities, who they were looking for adoptive homes for. And I thought, 'Hmmm, that could be interesting.' I had someone from the department come out and talk to me about what type of children they had, and whether or not we were likely to qualify to adopt. They all had disabilities. Yes, it was a free range from multiple profound disabilities through to Down syndrome, and I think a child who was blind. So it was the entire spectrum. They were all babies who had been surrendered at birth. I am only aware of one where the mother had intended before the birth to place the child for adoption anyway, and then went ahead with that decision. The rest of the families, as far as I know, were intending to have raised a healthy, happy child until the day it was delivered and they discovered that this wasn't what they were looking for. So I spoke to the people from Community Services and they gave me a bit of information about what it might be like, what some of the problems could be, what I was in for.

At this stage Helen introduced her family to the idea. They had grown up comfortable with the notion of adoption and it was the disability which was the issue. After deliberation, both her children, aged ten and fifteen, decided they were happy with the idea, but Helen's husband Colin was not.

Not to love a child that wasn't his, of course that wasn't a problem, but he was very doubtful about whether he could love a child with a disability. He then came back to me a couple of days later and asked to be able to meet a family who had a child with Down syndrome.

The family had already decided that if they did go ahead, a child with Down syndrome would suit them best.

The kids had said, 'If we're going to do this we want it to be someone who we can play with, who we can go out and do things with, because a child that is in a wheelchair — we can't do that.' So the Down syndrome seemed to me to be the logical way to go. And Family Services were quite happy for us to say, 'This type of child would suit our family best,' or 'I couldn't possibly cope with this one but I think I could cope with that one.' They were I think probably more confident that it would work if we were actually being open enough to say, 'I don't think I could handle that one.' Some of the children they had to place had really really profound disability. They would have been very difficult.

In Western Australia, the process of adopting children with disabilities is the same as for those without. It can take months, and involves the prospective parents in a series of interviews on numerous topics, usually with social workers. After the child is placed in its new home, there may be one or two follow-up visits until the adoption is finalised, which can take a further year or so, but thereafter the child is effectively deemed to be the responsibility of the adoptive family and the department withdraws. Once the family's decision was made, things progressed smoothly and Damian joined the Golding family, to be followed in later years by Charlotte, then finally by Josie. Helen's only gripe was that even on the third time round, when the family was actually approached by the department and asked to adopt, they still had to go through the whole process of screening.

Iris Fisher and her husband formally fostered their own granddaughter, not because the child had Down syndrome but because their daughter's own circumstances weren't conducive to caring for a child. The young mother herself had actually been adopted by the couple as a baby in the 1960s.

When I adopted Sally, children with disabilities weren't allowed out into the community. You could only adopt perfect babies. As a matter of fact, Sally was three and a half months; she was held back because she had sticky eyes and they wanted to make sure there wasn't any malformation or lasting problems. Any child with any problems that way was put in a home. So you only adopted 'perfect health' children.

Nowadays, few 'perfect health' Australian children without disabilities are available for adoption and families who do adopt are more likely to adopt a child 'with a difference' — a child from China or Korea, or perhaps a child with a disability. Within Australia there are few such children available for adoption, but in the United States, where both adoption and migration laws make the process far simpler for couples wanting to adopt a child from overseas, with or without a disability, the situation is very different. The websites of organisations such as Rainbowkids and Reece's Rainbow list any number of children with Down syndrome available for adoption from all over the world. Indeed the children are pictured by country of origin and one can choose from a veritable international smorgasbord. My first response to this approach was, it's like choosing puppies from an animal shelter site. On further reflection though, the future awaiting some of these children, especially those in orphanages in parts of Eastern Europe, was not one I would wish upon a dog.

The paucity of children available for adoption from within the United States underlines the fact that there, as in Australia, relinquishing an unwanted child for adoption is infinitely less common than terminating a pregnancy following prenatal diagnosis of a disability. Addressing this, the right-to-life oriented International Down Syndrome Coalition for

Life (IDSC for Life) advocates explicitly for children with Down syndrome 'in the womb and in the room'. As well as campaigning against the ninety per cent (or nine-out-of-ten, as the IDSC for Life puts it) abortion rate which prevails in the United States for pregnancies with Down syndrome diagnosed prenatally, it also offers advice and counselling for those who wish to relinquish, and provides links to organisations which support adoption. The IDSC for Life position is that, even if a family itself does not wish to raise a child with Down syndrome, there is no need to deny that child life or other families the opportunity to parent, and that the promotion of alternatives to abortion might help some people respond differently to a prenatal diagnosis of Down syndrome.[33]

Yet it appears that, not much more than a long generation after parents accepted institutionalisation of their children (for the sake of the child, it was said, and for the greater good of the family), western societies have moved very firmly to a position where the preferred alternative to raising a child with Down syndrome is termination of the pregnancy. The process has been facilitated by the now almost universal availability of prenatal screening and diagnosis, and the subsequent availability of abortion.

In the United States the debate on this subject, though not the abortion rate, has progressed further than in Australia. In September 2008 the federal *Prenatally and Postnatally Diagnosed Conditions Awareness Act* was passed.[34] It requires that parents who receive a diagnosis of a condition such as Down syndrome be provided with current information about the condition and given access to support networks and other services. Among its supporters the late Senator Ted Kennedy argued that 'access to the best support and information about the condition, and the quality of life for a child born with that condition, can make all the difference to a woman trying to make an informed and difficult decision.'[35] Interestingly, the lead-up to the Act brought together both pro-life and pro-choice advocates, with the focus on informed consent seen as critical by both camps.

The statistics on abortion give a very clear snapshot of what is happening in Western Australia. As more older women have more babies, the number of pregnancies with Down syndrome increases, yet the number of births of babies with Down syndrome has not increased, indicating that a higher proportion of pregnancies where Down syndrome is present end in termination.

At the same time as more older women are having more babies, the antenatal tests available have become more sophisticated and more accurate in indicating Down syndrome. Antenatal screening for conditions such as Down syndrome first became available in Australia in the early 1980s, at which point the only test available was amniocentesis, an invasive procedure which involves testing the amniotic fluid in the uterus at about eighteen weeks into the pregnancy. Subsequently chorionic villus sampling (CVS) was developed, a test which takes cells from the placenta itself. Despite some initial problems associated with damage to foetal limbs, medical practitioners preferred this test because it could be performed earlier in a pregnancy and consequently a woman could be offered an earlier term abortion. Typically, these two invasive diagnostic procedures involve some risk of miscarriage and formerly a woman was not advised to consider such testing unless she was of 'advanced maternal age' — until the 1990s defined as aged forty or over; now mid thirties and over.

While these tests established the presence of foetuses with Down syndrome in older women, Down syndrome in pregnancies among younger women — the group which still had by far the majority of babies and the majority of babies with the condition — remained undetected. Subsequently, less invasive screening tests were introduced and these are now performed on most pregnant Western Australian women irrespective of age as part of the normal suite of pregnancy-associated blood tests and ultrasound for things such as iron levels, rubella and blood group. Two tests are now generally available: triple test screening (TTS), which is undertaken in the second trimester, was introduced in Western Australia in the early 1990s, and first trimester pregnancy screening (FTS), which has generally available since 1999–2000.[36]

FTS involves a blood test ideally at week ten of the pregnancy, followed by an ultrasound at week twelve. The specialised ultrasound enables a measurement of the thickness or translucency of the baby's neck (the nuchal fold) and this result taken in conjunction with the mother's age and the results of the blood test, are used to calculate a likelihood of Down syndrome. Should a woman miss this window, or if she lives in regional Western Australia where the specialised ultrasound is not available, then the TTS is available between 15 and 18 weeks of pregnancy. It is regarded as less accurate than the FTS. These blood tests are described as 'screening' rather than 'diagnostic', meaning they cannot diagnose whether or not Down syndrome is present, but simply provide statistics on likelihood. Should the chance of Down syndrome (or other detectable conditions) be high, a woman will normally be offered further diagnostic testing in the form of CVS or amniocentesis, depending on the stage of the pregnancy.

In 2004, 70 per cent of pregnant Western Australian women underwent first or second trimester screening. Only in South Australia (80 per cent) is the screening rate higher, while rates elsewhere range from 17 per cent in the Northern Territory to 39 per cent in Queensland, 47 per cent in Tasmania, 54 per cent in Victoria, 57 per cent in the ACT, and 60 per cent in New South Wales.[37] The introduction of these screening tests has meant that more pregnancies with Down syndrome are now diagnosed prenatally across the whole maternal age range. According to the WA Birth Defects Registry the number of births of children with Down syndrome in Western Australia has remained fairly consistent at 1 in 1000 over the last few years, indicating a rise in the rate of terminations, which is presently about 90 per cent following prenatal diagnosis.

In theory a woman would be advised of the significance of any screening test she is having. A pamphlet produced by one of the state's leading diagnostic pathologists advises: 'Before undergoing this test it is very important you have discussed this testing procedure with your doctor.'[38] Similarly, the offer of further tests should be made neutrally in an atmosphere of informed consent, or in conjunction with specialist genetic counselling. However, this is not always the case in practice, a fact which has been the focus of considerable research, debate and anger, nationally and internationally.[39]

Jennifer Ravi's first daughter Amber, who was born in Perth in 1992, has Down syndrome. When Jennifer was expecting her second child in 1994 she had what she thought of as 'the usual' series of blood tests but was not in any way counselled or even advised that one was a screening test for Down syndrome. Consequently Jennifer was alarmed to be phoned at work late on a Friday afternoon by the doctor's receptionist, to be told that there seemed to be something 'wrong' with the baby. Not able to speak to her doctor, she spent the weekend miserably wondering what the chances were of having two children with Down syndrome. She was also angry. She had not sought this information, had not knowingly consented to having the test undertaken, and did

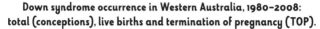

Down syndrome occurrence in Western Australia, 1980–2008: total (conceptions), live births and termination of pregnancy (TOP).

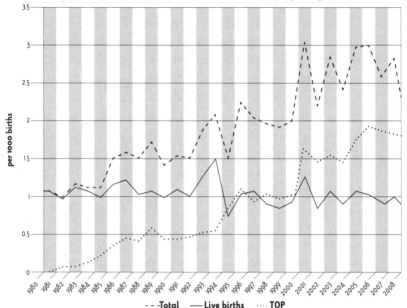

This figure illustrates that the occurrence of Down syndrome in pregnancies (births plus terminations) and the rate of terminations have both increased steadily since 1980. The impact of the introduction of screening tests from the mid 1990s is very clear. From this point, the number of babies born with Down syndrome falls below the number of pregnancies resulting in a termination.

Between 2004 and 2008 terminations occurred in 90 per cent of pregnancies where Down syndrome was diagnosed prenatally. Of all pregnancies where Down syndrome was present, 62 per cent resulted in a termination. The 38 per cent of pregnancies which resulted in the birth of a baby with Down syndrome comprised those diagnosed prenatally and those where there was no prenatal diagnosis. The rate of Down syndrome in live births in Western Australia has remained around 1 per 1000 for many years.

Source: C. Bower, E. Rudy, A. Callaghan, J. Quick, P. Cosgrove, N. Nassar, Report of the Birth Defects Registry of Western Australia 1980–2008, Perth, King Edward Memorial Hospital, December 2009, Number 16.

not wish to have it. Believing that her second child also had Down syndrome did not affect her attitude to the viability of the pregnancy, and she refused her doctor's suggestion that she have further diagnostic testing, on the grounds that it was invasive and in any case would not change her intentions regarding the pregnancy. But she remained upset that the information had been obtained without her informed consent. In fact when her daughter was born, to Jennifer's shock the child did *not* have Down syndrome. Hers was a case where inaccurate information imparted by the screening test robbed her of peace of mind during the pregnancy and did not alter the outcome.[40]

Since the introduction of enhanced screening procedures, the rate of abortion has risen and the proportion of children born with Down syndrome has fallen, leading some commentators, such as Canadian bioethicist Margaret Somerville, to label screening as a 'search and destroy' mission amounting to eugenics.[41] Consequently there has been a significant amount of research into the issues associated with decision-making in this sphere, largely around the role of doctors in counselling patients, in terms of both undergoing screening tests in the first place and explaining what they mean. A major international study showed the complexity of the situation.[42] Some women, for example, were not offered a choice in terms of prenatal screening, whereas others found the need to make a choice in itself a source of confusion and anxiety. While research has generally focused on the feelings of the women involved, the attitudes of doctors, including their own personal values, and of partners, were also important influences on the counselling process and the outcomes.

The assumption that women would automatically move to terminate a pregnancy if there was evidence of a chromosomal abnormality might seem a reasonable one given the statistics on terminations, but it is certainly not universally true. For example, when Julia Anderson and her politician husband John (later leader of the National Party and deputy prime minister of Australia) learned in 1997 that their unborn child had Down syndrome, they elected to continue with the pregnancy, though Julia was told she was the only one of four women similarly diagnosed that week who did so.[43] A complex array of factors including age of the parents involved and likelihood of having another baby in the future, religion, cultural and personal values, social pressure, attitude to disability generally, all influence the decision, but informed and up to date knowledge of the condition is also critical. A recent Western Australian scientific study makes this point very clearly. The health and longevity prospects for children with Down syndrome born today are excellent, a fact which the study's authors suggest should be pointed out to parents when counselling them on their possible response to a positive screening diagnosis.[44] Too often unfortunately, counselling is undertaken by a woman's GP, who may be regrettably ignorant of the implications of conditions such as Down syndrome. This theme is explored in the subsequent chapter.

Doctors alone cannot be held responsible for the rise in the statistics on abortion, but anecdotal evidence suggests they seldom play a neutral role. Perth woman Carla Zwetsloot, for example, told the West Australian in 2008 about the counselling she was given by her midwife and obstetrician once she found that the baby she was carrying had Down syndrome. 'They quietly took me aside and said, "People don't keep them, they terminate them."'[45] Though she decided not to do what other people did, statistics tell us she was in a minority. Whether people are swayed by such medical counselling or whether this would have been their response anyway is more difficult to measure.

Jude Lawrence's second child Laura had Down syndrome. She fell pregnant again soon after Laura was born and she and her partner Luke Middleton decided they wanted to know whether their next child had Down syndrome as well. After genetic counselling, where the likelihood of having a baby with Down syndrome or another condition was discussed, Jude opted to have a CVS at a major Perth maternity hospital. On the day of the procedure she felt ill-prepared and shared her anxieties and doubts about whether she even wanted to be there with the nurse who was attending her. The nurse, it seemed, had a sister with Down syndrome, who had died, and she was very sure what Jude's position should be: 'Well, you've got a little girl with Down syndrome and of course you love her, but you wouldn't want another one, would you!' To cap it off, as Jude lay waiting for the procedure, the attending doctor struck up a conversation after perusing her notes. 'One child with Down syndrome already? Well, we can do nothing about the past, but we can do everything about the future!'

The godlike assumption from doctors that they know best what patients (should) feel and how they should act, can leave parents with little room for objective reflection. Some doctors go even further than this. Jackie Softly spent a number of years working at the Down Syndrome Association office in Perth and had spoken to many parents about doctors' attitudes to prenatal screening.

I've heard some people say, 'My doctor will only do testing for me if I agree to terminate if there is a problem,' and I just think that is the height of lack of understanding and arrogance; to say to someone, before they even have the test, that 'You must assure me that you will terminate.' I can't understand that, because I don't honestly know how you could ever make any sort of a decision until you've got the results.[46]

Virginia Robb also decided not to have diagnostic screening for the pregnancy following the birth of her daughter Georgia, who has Down syndrome, and was similarly shocked by one doctor's attitude to her decision. Incidentally, this was a doctor who worked in the disability sector.

I got blasted by the doctor at Disability Services. I took Georgia there for the general medical check-up and I must have told the doctor I was pregnant, and she just tore strips off me and told me that I could have another child with Down syndrome and I was selfish and di-da di-da. I came home, I was a mess. I actually put in a grievance against her and got an apology. Because it was none of her business. But I know that other people had complained about her as well, she used to tell people that they should put their child on the pill when they were twelve and all kinds of things like that. So I don't think she was the right person to be there.

Fortunately, this position is not universal among medical practitioners, some of whom even have children with Down syndrome themselves. Brenda Harvey's experience in Albany, a smaller regional centre in the south-west of the state, was entirely different and much more positive. She was forty when she fell pregnant with her third child Grace in 1991.

During the pregnancy somebody said to me, 'Have you had any tests?' And I thought, 'Well, should I?' And I took a long time to decide about that. Initially, I thought, 'No, no. I don't need to do that.' But then I did decide to have it, because I thought, 'Well, if something was terribly, terribly wrong, I don't think I would be able to cope with it,' and so I decided to do the test, an amniocentesis. And I was actually on the table and they were just about to put the needle into my tummy and I changed my mind! The reason was that they had the ultrasound on, and on the screen I saw — a baby, a fully formed baby — and as soon as I saw that, the possibility of aborting it was, you know, I just didn't want that to happen. It was like, in every cell in my body, there were bells ringing saying, 'No, no, no, no, don't do this!' So I asked them to stop, and they were very, very good about it, and they did stop. And they asked me, did I want to have time to think about it? And so I went back to the room where they gave me time.

I can't rightly remember now exactly what was said, but I do know there was *no* pressure put on me at all. What I realised was that previously, I felt that I wasn't strong enough to cope if anything was wrong, but now I realised I would be strong enough, that even if I did the test and they told me that there was something wrong with the child, I couldn't abort it. And as soon as it was clear in my own head that, no, I wouldn't do that anyway, then there was no point in having the test. And so I went away feeling very clear and relieved and very positive again, and I never ever thought about it from that moment onwards.

After Grace was born, the certainty that this had been the right decision remained with Brenda, who said, 'I didn't even think about it. Didn't even question it. There was no "I wished I'd known": none of that.'

For medical practitioners, fear of litigation may be a factor behind an aggressive approach towards the question of termination, as suggested in 2008 in discussion focused on the US *Prenatally and Postnatally Diagnosed Conditions Awareness Act*. In Australia there have been a number of court cases associated with the concept of 'wrongful life' in which it is argued that the defendant medical practitioner does not cause the disability but, rather, fails to avert it.

In response to two separate cases, the Australian High Court decided in 2006 that there were no grounds for compensation on the basis of alleged 'wrongful life' because it could not be shown that the child's alternative position — not being alive — was preferable to being alive, with judges arguing that disability was not the sole determinant of a person's quality of life.[47] While disability activists applauded this decision, doctors also undoubtedly heaved a sigh of relief. In France in 2002, a similar decision was effectively forced upon the French courts when protesting doctors refused to undertake any further prenatal screening after courts had found in favour of a child with Down syndrome who had successfully sued a doctor for having failed to advise its parents of the possibility of the condition.[48] Yet in August 2009, a New South Wales couple sued the Mercy Hospital in Sydney because they 'ought to have told them' to have more tests for Down syndrome; the woman had evidently had an ultrasound but had not realised this was not foolproof in ruling out Down syndrome and was apparently not counselled regarding the availability of further diagnostic testing.[49] The case was set for mediation in 2010.

Why would you want to know whether your child had Down syndrome if you didn't intend to do anything about it? For some parents, for the same reason as wanting to know the gender of a child: to prepare themselves mentally. Among the families I spoke to, the desire to know was often heightened in pregnancies following the birth of a child with Down syndrome but there was no consensus on how a family would respond. In many cases, the birth of that first child sometimes changed attitudes to antenatal screening deeply and confusingly. Parents didn't necessarily know what they would do, but still they wanted that information. Discussion and decision-making could come later. Luke Middleton and partner Jude Lawrence, for example, had elected not to discuss the topic until they had a test result.

Luke: The big question which I always asked myself was, what would we have done if the child had Down syndrome? I persuaded myself that we would have had her, had two kids with Down syndrome. I've given a few talks about this to people, and people always ask me this question, and I say that I would like to have thought that we would have kept the child.

Jan: You would 'like to have thought' — how do you mean?

Luke: Yes. Well I'm pretty sure that we would have kept the child, in fact I'm positive that we would have kept the child; but there's always this moment where you think, perhaps you mightn't have. But I know it would have been a very hard decision.

After their first child was born with Down syndrome, Richard and Beth Gregson decided they wanted to know whether their next child would also have the condition, but they too baulked at fully exploring their feelings about how to deal with that possibility until it became reality.

We both wanted to have tests, as soon as we found out. We really did want to have the tests. We wanted to know whether we were going to have the double trouble of having two Downs rather than one. So, we had some tests done and this time we had an actual proper chromosome test done because we wanted to be certain. Beth is forty and so you have to bear that in mind as well. We did talk a little bit about how we might react to another Downs child, though probably not as much as what we could or should have, but personally I found it, I think Beth did too, a little bit difficult talking in depth about it. I think because we knew that we would know anyway, one way or the other, so we copped out a little bit, you know, we won't necessarily have to go through the whole process of what we would do if it was. All we knew was that it would add additional pressure to the family, having another one. Having been through so much and worked so hard with Jordan and him still being young, and having another one on top of it this late in our lives, it would've been difficult. We both knew it would be difficult. And that is why we wanted the tests and that is why we did talk about it briefly but we didn't focus too much on it.

Others though felt no need to know at all.[50] The Brookton family, for instance, had no wish to screen for Down syndrome in the pregnancy following the birth of their son with Down syndrome. As Keith said, 'Well if we had another kid with Down syndrome, we had another kid with Down syndrome.'

For Karen Langley and Paolo da Silva, their second pregnancy after the birth of Shannon was not planned, but it was not wholly unexpected and certainly not unwelcome. They opted for genetic counselling and antenatal testing. But, unlike those parents who chose not to discuss possible outcomes and consequences till they had the test results, circumstances compelled Karen and Paolo to make a decision well ahead of the testing.

At the time that I discovered I was pregnant we were planning to go to the Himalayas as a family. And we would have been there at just about the time when I would have had to have amniocentesis and you are obviously not going to have that in the Himalayas. So Paolo went, and I went to my parents. And the upshot of that was we basically had to decide in advance what we thought we might do if this were positive. We discussed it in the context of, if the amniocentesis comes through and we are expecting another baby with Down syndrome, we'd have a termination. Because we can do *one* with special needs; but *two* with special needs, we wouldn't have the time for either of them that we would want, and to go through all that stuff with heart surgery possibly and all that again, we just didn't want to do it ...

So, we decided that if we were expecting another child with a genetic problem, I would terminate the pregnancy, and that this would be without further discussion, because it was practically impossible to get a phone call through at that time to the Himalayas anyway. So there was really no room for either of us to be saying, 'Oh well, we will say this now but we might change our minds later.' No matter what either of us felt, we weren't going back on it. And in retrospect, both of us admitted to the other afterwards that we had actually realised that we had made the wrong decision! Had the amniocentesis shown there was another baby with a genetic defect, we had both decided that we didn't care. But we'd made this pact that we weren't going to change anything, so it would have been a complete disaster, because I mean, I would have terminated a pregnancy that both of us actually wanted! So fortunately, everything was okay.

Loretta Muller and Andrew Danes were also clear that they would have had a termination if they found they were expecting a second child with Down syndrome. Like some other families, their subsequent pregnancy was a deliberate decision made as a consequence of their first child's disability, and having a second child with a disability was not part of that plan.

We thought about whether it was better to just have *him* and be able to offer him more attention, or whether we should have a brother or a sister to keep him company, and perhaps he could learn off them, and perhaps they could help him and in the long term, when we're not around then they would be around to help look after him when he's older. So we decided we would have another one and we did, very quickly. But when I was pregnant with Sarah I chose to have a CVS and there were issues with that too, because before we had it done we felt like we had to decide what would happen if we got a result that said this child has a disability as well. We decided that if that was the case we would terminate the pregnancy. We didn't think it was fair to any of us in the family to have another child with a disability. (Loretta Muller)

An unwelcome complication for some families, but particularly for mothers, was the intervention of other women who felt they had some right to question or advise. Wendy Brookton saw her own position on prenatal testing as an ethical stance and expressed some anger at the attitudes of some of her friends when they learned she wasn't intending to have screening for a subsequent pregnancy. While she didn't tell them how offensive she found their attitude, she 'certainly shied away from them.'

A few said, 'Oh I can't believe you're ...' In other words they didn't think that Mark was a worthwhile person. They made their moral choice, I'll make mine, which is not to encourage those sorts of people to make judgements on other people.

Britt Canning was also extremely sensitive to the perceived implications of her decision to have prenatal testing in the pregnancy following the birth of her son with Down syndrome, to the point where she and her husband decided on a strategy to head off unwanted questions.

> I felt it was such a complex decision for me to make that I didn't want others to know, because they couldn't take into account all those complexities. For me it wasn't a reflection on Jack, and yet I felt that if people knew I was going to have a test they would see that as me not accepting him. It wasn't. It was separate to Jack completely. I needed to be reassured. So we decided our standard line would be, if someone said, 'Are you having tests?' we would say, 'Well, we have discussed it and have decided to keep that between ourselves.' Basically nicely saying, 'Mind your own business' ... I felt it was really presumptuous of people to even ask. One woman [herself the mother of a child with Down syndrome] was quite aggressive about it and when I gave my standard line, she was saying, 'Well, why don't you tell us?' and I said, 'Well, I don't want to, I don't want to be influenced by anybody else.' She came out and said, 'If you have a test then it means you don't accept this child.' She was saying *she* could never have a test, it would be an awful thing for her own child. And I thought, well, none of your business. But then my *good* friends with children with Down syndrome never asked.

As she outlined in a subsequent interview, by the time she was pregnant with her third child in 2001 Britt had had two babies (one with Down syndrome) and two miscarriages, so by that stage she had become more concerned about the prospect of a further miscarriage than disability. On that basis, she said, 'I decided just to go ahead and try not to worry.'

The decision is certainly a more complicated one for people who already have a child with Down syndrome. Heather

Burton thought along the same lines as Britt Canning had done about the decision and how she might respond to the outcome.

I thought very long and hard about it, because on the one hand I felt that if I had found out that I was having another child with Downs and I terminated it, that that would be totally discrediting who Lucy is, and saying that who she is, is not okay. So I grappled and I still grapple with that. But the other issue I felt was, I've got my child with a disability and I really don't know that it would feel right for us to have another one in terms of our family and how we cope or don't cope. Fortunately I didn't have to make the decision, so I still don't really know what I would have done.

I just think when so many of my friends would say, 'Oh have you had your amnio yet?' as if it's the easiest thing in the world, I would always sit there thinking, 'You have no idea what you're talking about,' because unless you really have to face that decision it's not something you just do. It's huge, you're talking life and death.

The Webbs were divided in their views on how they would have responded to a subsequent pregnancy with Down syndrome following the birth of their daughter Nicola in 1980. Steph was unequivocal but her husband Paul was much more ambivalent.

Steph: I know if I would have had another child with a disability I definitely would have had it terminated because I just think, well I've already had Nicola, I'm going to have to look after her, I would not be able to look after two with a disability and it wouldn't be fair to Nicola. So yes, I had the amnio and yes, everything was fine. The doctor said, 'Well the chances of Down syndrome again are slim.' But I said I wanted it done just to be sure. I didn't want another child with a disability because it was hard going.

Jan: And the decision was made before you had the test?

Steph: Oh definitely, yes. Otherwise I wouldn't have had the test.

Paul: If they'd have asked us before Nicola was born, saying, 'Hey she's Down syndrome,' for sure we would say, 'Oh, we'll terminate.' But *after* having a child with Down syndrome, I doubt very much that I would. Yes, it would be a very hard decision to make today knowing what Down syndrome can be — but boy, there's a lot of worse things out there than Down syndrome.

Steph: No, I definitely would have had it terminated.

Jan (to Paul): And you would have found it harder perhaps?

Paul: Oh, you see it's not my problem, is it?

Jan: So you saw it as Steph's decision?

Paul: Oh of course. I mean if anyone should take any credit for what Nicola is or isn't, it's Steph, because of all the work she's put in.

Pamela Franklin also saw the decision about prenatal testing and its consequences as the mother's. She was 'ten days off forty' when her daughter was born in 1984.

I was offered an amnio by my doctor, because of my age. But I didn't want one because I wouldn't have had an abortion anyway. It was not a decision that was hard to make. I am a Catholic and abortion certainly goes against that religion, but I am against it whether or not I am a Catholic. But my husband hasn't got a religious background, which I think is probably important. He always had a philosophy that kids with disabilities, in nature they'd get left by the wayside and they wouldn't survive; and we are not going to be able to look after all the people who need looking after. We had always argued about things like that because he basically has a different philosophy on humanity than I do. And I suppose I hadn't discussed amnio with him. But I doubt whether he would've wanted me to have an abortion. Put it this way, if I had told him and he *had* wanted me to have an abortion, I don't think we would be married now. And the way it's turned out, the greatest fan Catherine's got is her dad.

Parental age is another complicating factor. I spoke to my brother about prenatal diagnosis when he was contemplating starting a family later in life. He was nearly fifty, his partner over forty, and their position was very clear: as older parents, knowingly taking on responsibility for a child who was unlikely to be independent by the age of about twenty was not an option.

Even a prenatal 'all clear' was not enough to allay all concerns about a baby's health and few if any parents remembered experiencing anxiety-free pregnancies after the birth of a child with Down syndrome, regardless of their position on prenatal testing. Having become part of the disability world, parents were usually more sensitive to the possibility that things don't always work out the way one might expect or hope. At the time I interviewed Richard Gregson, he and his wife Beth were expecting their third child.

Well the tests showed that the baby doesn't have Down syndrome, but it doesn't necessarily mean it is going to be a perfectly healthy baby. It could have other problems.

Trish Weston had remained similarly anxious about her new babies' health despite prenatal testing for two subsequent pregnancies.

I had some feeling of relief when the tests came back but that certainly didn't make me feel that everything was going to be fine. I still didn't feel that we were out of the woods, as it were, and I knew by then, having been to Irrabeena, that there were a lot of other things that this baby could have that you could never pick up with any sort of prenatal diagnosis; and having that awareness made me realise that, well, you know, we can't relax just yet. And I think I was a bit obsessive about this. I told the obstetrician that as soon as this baby was born I wanted a paediatrician to come in, and not the one that we had last time, thank you, and do a really thorough check. And I did that with Amy too. I was so obsessed and so keen to know that everything would be just fine — straightaway! So I wasn't prepared to sort of say, 'Oh, phew, the tests have come back negative. Everything's fine now. We can just relax.' I didn't feel that way.

I was not able to interview families who had terminated a pregnancy following a diagnosis of Down syndrome, but I did speak to some who knew their child had Down syndrome before it was born. Malcolm Barnes and his wife Kerry were about to embark on an IVF program in 2005 when to their delight, they discovered that thirty-seven year old Kerry was already pregnant. As all the scans and screening tests indicated a low likelihood of genetic problems, they 'opted not to take the risk' of diagnostic screening. But for the need to reduce the level of amniotic fluid for medical reasons, they would have remained unaware that their child had Down syndrome until his birth. When this fluid was drained off, however, subsequent testing — of which the couple thought nothing — led to the discovery that their unborn son had Down syndrome, information which caused them all the pain, grief and emotion experienced by parents when they receive such news at birth.

They considered the options, with termination foremost in their minds. The pregnancy was too far advanced for an 'easy legal termination' so the couple appealed to a medical panel for permission, which was denied. However, once they understood what such a late termination would have entailed — injecting the child *in utero* and effectively killing it, then delivering the dead baby normally and even, as they said, having a funeral — they felt that continuing with the pregnancy was the correct decision.

> Had we known *very* early on, say four to twelve weeks in, we would have terminated, which is a major travesty in my opinion, now I know what I know!

> Knowing later on and not having alternatives I think is better, as you have time to educate and prepare yourselves. This also allows the parents to accept the child before birth, which I believe is a bonus.

Like many parents, Malcolm's views on early termination changed significantly once his son was born. Today (aged three) their son is 'a bright, happy and independent little boy who can talk, walk, run, count and sign — not bad eh?'

Another couple also found out about their daughter's Down syndrome as a result of medical intervention. Virginia Robb was on the pill when she conceived and in many ways considered her pregnancy a miracle, having been told after her second child was born that she couldn't have any more children because of her severe rhesus condition. After accidentally falling pregnant however, she learned that technology had advanced to the point where intra-uterine blood transfusions were possible.

The pregnancy demanded constant monitoring and medical intervention at King Edward Memorial Hospital, with the unborn baby requiring four transfusions. It was after one of those, when Virginia was twenty-four weeks pregnant, that they found out the baby had Down syndrome. The doctor saw the thickening of the neck, the nuchal fold, and said, 'Oh, might just test and see if it's Down syndrome.'

Virginia was a teacher in her thirties when she fell pregnant with Georgia, and had been advised to consider diagnostic testing.

> I opted not to because I wouldn't have terminated anyway, so I figured that the less invasion and interference I could do with the better, because I knew that rhesus was pretty risky anyway.

As a Catholic she was also opposed to termination on religious grounds, and her husband, a non-Catholic, supported her in her decision to continue with the pregnancy once the Down syndrome was discovered. Like Malcolm and Kerry, the couple went through the whole process of pain and disbelief and of informing friends and family.

> I was working and I got a phone call at work in the middle of a lesson saying, 'Got the results back; oh, by the way your child has Down syndrome.' So that was a bit of a shock. We did know they were testing for it. It's just that was a bit hard in the middle of a working day, because I had to go back into my class ...

> There was nothing we could do about it anyway. I mean, I'd felt her kicking and moving and I couldn't. Catholic beliefs totally to one side I just wouldn't have been able to do it. I was six months pregnant basically. I was surprised I was

even offered a termination to be honest, but I guess they have to offer you ...

We were in shock really and so we went down to Fremantle and there was some match racing, sailing. And we saw about seven people with Down syndrome! It's like when you get a red car — they're everywhere! We couldn't believe it. I think we just sat and contemplated. I suppose all the things that go through your head are all those things that you're afraid of, like what happens when we get old, what's she going to be like when she's a teenager. It wasn't even the birth, it wasn't even all the risks associated with the current health problems; I was projecting into the future, which I guess is normal.

But in hindsight I am really glad we knew because what we actually did, when we look back, we grieved for the child that we thought we were going to have, so we got through our grieving, and by the time she was born we just celebrated her birth. She was an emergency caesarean as well, so we were just grateful that she was alive. Whereas obviously people who don't find out till the child's born ... I think we were lucky, I really do, because we'd got through all those emotions.

Emily Howard was twenty-eight when her son Joseph was born in 2008. She had testing early in the pregnancy — a blood test and an associated scan and nuchal fold measurement — which suggested she was at high risk of having a child with Down syndrome, but even so, she felt it really wasn't going to happen. In fact disability had not crossed her mind when she fell pregnant. Like many others, she assumed 'those kinds of things' didn't happen to people like her. Her view of children with Down syndrome was that they were the last-born in big Catholic families, always with older mothers: not her profile at all! Though she had known the blood test was used for screening for Down syndrome, she had no idea of the significance of the associated scan, and recalled that it was presented to her not as part of a screening procedure but as an opportunity to take home some great video footage of her unborn baby.

After the initial screening result, the decision to have follow-up diagnostic screening was a fraught one for her and her husband Ben. They had already decided that, even if there was a diagnosis of Down syndrome, they would continue with the pregnancy. So why have the test? While Emily said she did not actually feel 'pressured' by her obstetrician, he had counselled her strongly to go ahead with it in view of the screening results, and she too had started to become anxious and felt that she really wanted confirmation that everything was fine. And if not, she laughed, 'I had what turned out to be a completely unrealistic expectation that this cavalry comes and helps you!'

Emily's obstetrician was based in a big private hospital in Perth which for religious and ethical reasons does not permit the performance of the sorts of diagnostic and screening procedures her doctor prescribed, so, like all his patients, she was sent back across the road to the private radiology practice where she had had her earlier testing. The risk of miscarriage with the recommended CVS was high and, in view of Emily's firm belief that there was nothing wrong, she and her husband considered the risk unacceptable, so they opted for an amniocentesis. A few days later she got a phone call from her obstetrician's nurse, who announced, 'Honey, you've got a Downs on board.'

For Emily that was where the nightmare began, but ironically, this had little to do with the diagnosis. The news was a shock but did not change her attitude to the pregnancy.

Faced with the new reality though, her husband was a little less sure about whether he could take this on. A doctor himself, he did some thorough medical homework, confronted the worst the condition could offer and agreed with Emily that they should continue with the pregnancy. This must have been a worrying time for her though, as one of the other things she had been told by her obstetrician's nurse, when Emily said she wanted to continue with the pregnancy, was, '*You* might feel that way but in five years time your husband will have had enough and he'll leave you.'

As part of the process of information gathering, Emily rang her obstetrician's office, as a matter of theoretical interest, to find out exactly what would happen if she opted for a termination, and they were able to tell her a great deal about the process, which would take place at another hospital, and about all the available support and counselling.

Now satisfied that this was definitely *not* the way she wanted to go, Emily recalled saying, 'Okay, now I'm ready for the spiel,' expectantly awaiting information on what it meant to have a pregnancy and a baby with Down syndrome. The response from her obstetrician's rooms was shock: '"I don't know what to tell you! No one here has ever gone ahead!" I had to realise that I was in the abnormal group and they only dealt with the normal there.' To Emily's dismay, her baby was presented to her almost as a foreign object in her body.

'Get it out of my body' — I got the impression that that was how I was supposed to be feeling, but I didn't … From that moment things started to crumble for me because I realised that I was on my own and there was no cavalry coming.

The obstetrician himself was a little taken aback at their decision, and joked 'he would have to brush up on his text books.' Regrettably he didn't. When Emily's baby Joseph was born, it was immediately apparent that he had duodenal atresia, a condition with a fairly high correlation with Down syndrome, in which the baby's duodenum has not developed properly and the contents of its stomach cannot pass. This is usually diagnosed before birth and explained Emily's excess fluid during the pregnancy. After his birth, Joseph was taken straight to Princess Margaret Hospital for successful surgery. Subsequently they discovered that Joe also had a heart defect; it was corrected surgically a little later and as a result of his health conditions he had to be fed with a nasal gastric tube for the first six months of his life. None of this had been diagnosed during the pregnancy or discussed with Emily.

> I thought that that was the point of knowing, so that they could tell you these things so that you could be prepared, that he would have to have surgery, that he would have to have heart surgery, that he would have to be tube fed and all of those things.

So when her baby was born and was unexpectedly whisked away, she felt understandably 'robbed.'

Emily subsequently met other women whose babies had had duodenal atresia and all had been referred antenatally to a specialist. All those mothers had known beforehand that their babies would have to have bowel surgery when they were born and that they would have to go straight to Princess Margaret. Emily though felt that she and her husband and their complicated baby 'were just so inconvenient' to her obstetrician and his staff.

> The doctors and nursing staff just didn't seem to know what to do with us and we felt like aliens on their 'picture perfect' maternity ward. They seemed so put out that we didn't fit

into the ward's schedule because we were back and forth between the two hospitals so much.

Understandably, her response to the revelation of Joe's previously undiagnosed medical problems was enormous anger, not least when her obstetrician came to visit her hospital room and found her trying to express milk for tube-feeding her baby across town in Princess Margaret Hospital. 'All he wanted to know was, would it have changed our decision if we had known about Joe's other health issues' — which in the circumstances, perhaps he ought to have detected.

Getting up every three hours to express, going through all the effort and I was *still* having a doctor say to me, do you still want him? How many times do I have to tell you people?!

So despite the fact that she knew she was expecting a baby with Down syndrome, the birth was still full of unexpected emotion and surprises. Perhaps the biggest surprise for Emily though, having gone through the second half of her pregnancy expecting 'this baby that nobody could love but me,' was that her Joe was 'just gorgeous.'

Having a child with a disability doesn't automatically make you into a right to life campaigner, nor does it automatically make you a terminator, but it almost always makes the decision about prenatal diagnosis for subsequent pregnancies more complex, and reflection on what might have been becomes more painful. Britt Canning did not have any prenatal testing while expecting her first child Jack (she was twenty-four at the time).

I think I would have had a termination. I think I would have because I didn't have any children. I think that back then, like a lot of people when they are having their first, that I still saw this baby as just an extension of Peter and me. I didn't really comprehend that this was a completely unique individual — a part of us but quite separate from us. And I think my ego would have taken a huge blow if I had found out I was carrying a 'faulty' child; that just wouldn't have been good enough, not perfect enough. I don't think it is something I would have done lightly but I think I probably would have.

Trish Weston reached much the same conclusion. She had had no testing done when she was expecting Will (she was aged twenty-nine), but after his birth she felt her position on termination shifted considerably.

I think that I would have felt quite differently if I had testing done before Will was born. I think the fact that I was having testing done *after* I had this child with Down syndrome who I love very much, influenced me hugely. I really do. If I'd had testing done for my first-born, I think that I would have just seen it as a Down syndrome baby rather than an individual. And I think Will being our first child too was a factor. Probably for people who've already got other kids and then maybe find out that the baby they're carrying has Down syndrome, it might be harder for them to reach a decision, because they have already experienced caring for a child, for their own child, and that I think would place a completely different complexion on the whole thing. I think that it's certainly influenced me. I think it might have been easier for me to contemplate a termination of a baby with Down syndrome if I'd known before Will was born. I do.

In all the families I interviewed and the many other families I know with a child with Down syndrome, I know of no one who has had a second child with Down syndrome, though research tells us there is a higher chance of having a second child with a condition such as Down syndrome after the birth of a first, particularly if the mother was younger when the first child was born.[51]

In the United States, Michael Bérubé, parent and author of one of the best books around on Down syndrome, *Life As We Know It*, couples condemnation of 'uncritical advocates of prenatal screening' with a demand for enhanced social inclusion. As he wrote recently, some of the choices we have made have led us to 'a bitter paradox — that even though we haven't begun to explore the ways in which we could include people with disabilities in our society, we devote precious time and resources to developing better ways of spotting them before they are born.'[52] However, he has copped a great deal of flak for remaining pro-choice.

Personally, my position on abortion has also been immeasurably complicated by the issue of disability. I now find it infinitely harder to accept than I once would have done that disability alone can provide sufficient grounds for a termination. When I recently heard a woman behind the counter at a pathologists saying to a client in queue, 'Oh, so you are here for the Down syndrome test?' it reminded me my daughter is an aberration society would rather be without; it told me that medical specialists and their staff who make such statements do so within the terms of a particular view of disability; and it suggested to me there is little chance of the client receiving unbiased information or counselling at that clinic, should she be carrying a baby with Down syndrome. Twenty years ago though, I could well have been the woman in the queue.

In 2008 the UK press gave some coverage to a BBC program, *Born with Down's*, which suggested a rise in the incidence of births of babies with Down syndrome, apparently indicating that more women were choosing not to terminate babies with Down syndrome after receiving the results of prenatal screening and testing. The story, picked up by outlets ranging from *Marie Claire* to *The Times*, was newsworthy because it seemed at odds with the common assumption that people expecting a child with Down syndrome would almost automatically choose to terminate the pregnancy.[53] The United Kingdom's national Down syndrome organisation enthusiastically attributed this seemingly surprising shift in attitudes to increasingly positive perceptions of people with Down syndrome. Yet this proved to be false optimism. A report released by the National Down Syndrome Cytogenetic Register in response to the BBC's story suggested the statistics had been misinterpreted; that 92 per cent of women in Britain who have an antenatal diagnosis of Down syndrome have the pregnancy terminated and that this figure has not changed since 1989.[54] While the British press was eager to promote a view that suggested social attitudes were changing, that their society was becoming more inclusive and welcoming, a warmer and cuddlier place all round, in reality there was a profound gulf between what the media purported to aspire to for their society and what people were prepared to accept in their own homes. The rate of termination in the United Kingdom, as in the United States and in Australia, remains uniformly high and constant.

One mother captured the issue all too clearly. Gushed over once too often by a well-meaning but unthinking member of the 'They're all such dear little things' school, she finally snapped back, 'So how come you don't want one then?' We still have no adequate answer to that question.

But, given the choice, some people do opt for Down syndrome. Claudia Mansour says, 'If it wasn't for them, I wouldn't be the person I am today. If I had my life to live again I would have *two* instead of one.' Helen Golding adopted three children with Down syndrome. Iris Fisher fostered her granddaughter.

> She was the apple of my eye. I could never replace Trudy and I just wish I could have another one. If I was younger, I would adopt again.

Emily Howard sees it a little differently though.

> I don't think it really was a choice. He was Joe, he was always Joe. Just that somebody told me he wasn't going to be like I thought, but he was always Joe. It's not like he changed, just our idea of what he was going to be.

> And when Emily gets asked, as she sometimes does, whether she knew Joe had Down syndrome before he was born, 'I feel proud to say, yeah, I did.'

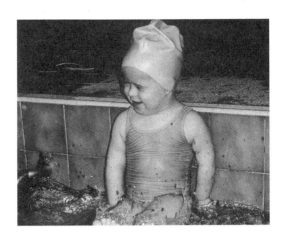

chapter 3

'IT'S NOT A DISEASE, YOU KNOW!':
DOWN SYNDROME AND MEDICAL ISSUES

'I guess the fact that we found out there were some tests
that we would have to have over and above a normal child
did cause us some anxiety.'
(Richard Gregson)

Down syndrome is not an illness, but most people don't know
that. People are often described as 'suffering from' Down
syndrome, as they would from flu or measles, and on first
diagnosis many parents ask whether it can be 'cured'. It's a
widespread and widely perpetuated misconception, and is
even officially promoted by the Australian government: a
person with Down syndrome applying to migrate to Australia
can be automatically refused permission on the grounds
that the individual, despite a perfect medical record, 'fails
to meet the health criteria' — as if Down syndrome signified

sickness, or a contagious disease.[55] Yet from the moment it is first recognised in a child, 'Down syndrome' is presented to parents bundled up in medical terminology. The condition, the diagnosis (which is usually delivered by a doctor or other health professional) and frequently the child itself, are 'medicalised'.

That being said, it is undeniable that Down syndrome has significant health implications for the individual, both negative and positive. Yet the enormous improvement in the health of people with Down syndrome over the past few decades shows very clearly that health is at least as dependent on initiatives in the public health area as it is on the disability itself. Changes in life expectancy, for example, are powerful evidence of shifts in both medical and social attitudes towards people with disabilities. In Western Australia in the period 1953 to 1979, some 80 per cent of people with Down syndrome died before they turned thirty, whereas in the period 1980 to 2005, only 39 per cent died by that age, meaning more than 60 per cent made it to their thirtieth birthday and almost half (48 per cent) attained the age of fifty. As well, the rate of death of people with Down syndrome in their first two to three years of life has plummeted since 1980.[56]

Statistically, children with Down syndrome are more likely than the rest of the population to experience cardiac, respiratory and gastrointestinal problems. They are also more prone to vision and hearing impairment or thyroid problems, though these are not life-threatening.

The turning point for the longevity of people with Down syndrome has really stemmed from two changes over the past three or four decades. The end of institutionalisation, and the associated increase in the practice of bringing up children with Down syndrome within the family, have made an enormous difference in terms of preventing premature death from respiratory-related causes such as bronchitis or pneumonia. These changes are part of a larger shift towards recognising people with Down syndrome as full members of society, with the same rights and expectations in terms of access to health care as others. At the same time, advances in cardiac surgery have enabled children with Down syndrome to undergo corrective surgery for life-threatening cardiac conditions. The heart is undoubtedly the Achilles heel for many people with Down syndrome — between 40 and 45 per cent of children born with Down syndrome are also born with heart defects.[57] In the past these often proved fatal and between them, cardiac and respiratory problems accounted for the premature deaths of the vast majority of people with Down syndrome.

Iris Fisher's granddaughter was among them.

In '89 we lost Trudy. Her death was very sudden, though in the February we had great hopes that an operation had become available that would perhaps have prolonged her life — another twenty years was the estimation, if she survived the operation — and we decided it was right for her to have that chance. They would need to do a catheterisation to see if she was fit enough for it and it was in that April that we were told that her lungs were too badly deteriorated. They couldn't even get through to do the catheterisation. That an operation wasn't feasible, and it was just a matter of time. Her heart was in such a bad condition, so much wrong with it. I was told there was nothing they could do. In September '89, she suddenly deteriorated. She went away on a Brownie camp and two weeks later she collapsed with her first fit, and within three days she was gone. They didn't resuscitate her or anything. They just didn't try, because they knew there was nothing they could do for her.

The situation has changed enormously since Trudy's death. But certainly in the 1980s the prospect of premature death seemed very real for new parents, as Trish Weston recalled.

When I rang my husband after I had the diagnosis confirmed by the obstetrician he'd fallen to pieces. He really didn't know anything about Down syndrome and his worry was actually, it turns out, not that Will had Down syndrome, but that he thought that people with Down syndrome died very young and that we were going to lose him. That was really his fear.

Highlighting the very positive aspect of changing life expectancy for people with Down syndrome would alleviate unnecessary anxiety for parents. From the moment of diagnosis though, they are often bombarded by information about negative health implications. Sometimes this is essential: the possibility of a congenital heart defect needs to be screened for as soon as possible after birth. But the information and the associated medicalisation of their newborn isn't always appreciated by already distraught parents like Karen Langley, who was trying desperately to cling to the positives following her daughter Shannon's birth.

We were presented with a file and a list of about 362 medical things that could go wrong and we just shut it again. And I don't think that we ever actually opened it again — we thought, at some point, that we might open it again later when we felt stronger, but I don't think we ever did!

The majority of people with Down syndrome do not experience particular ill health, but it is better to be on the lookout for the possibility of a condition such as thyroid or a heart defect with a view to dealing with it than to be unaware of its potential. Testing for defective hearing and vision are also part of this. Children with Down syndrome are more likely to have a defect in these areas, and are perhaps more vulnerable if such a condition is ignored. A child's capacity to draw on all its sensory skills can have a significant impact on development, especially with the contemporary emphasis on 'early intervention' and accelerated introduction to learning for children with learning delays.

> Jack can talk but his speech is very unclear. He did have glue ear quite badly and unfortunately the tests just weren't picking it up. So he was probably deaf till about the age of five. They couldn't get an accurate test because he wasn't very cooperative in the testing process, which is why no one had ever suggested that he have grommets. But in the end I pushed for him to have grommets because it seemed pretty obvious from his communication problems that he wasn't hearing properly. That did help, but I can't help thinking that we missed a pretty important window of opportunity there with him. (Britt Canning)

While professional monitoring is essential, parents are sometimes in a better position to judge from observation whether or not their child has a hearing problem. Helen Golding realised this on the brink of adopting her son Damian.

> When we actually got to the point of, 'Well, this is the child we think we would like you to have,' they also dropped on me that, 'We think he is profoundly deaf,' and I said, 'Well, I need to really think about that, because taking on a child with Down syndrome is one thing, taking on a child who is also profoundly deaf is something else again.' I met the foster mother and she said, 'He can hear; it's people in there that did the tests that are the problem, not him.' So the

foster mother and I decided that we would see a specialist who said, 'This child can hear. I can't tell you how good his hearing is, but he can hear.' Damian has this happy knack, whenever he was put into an unusual situation, of switching off entirely — he is still capable of doing that at the age of sixteen. And because they were getting no response they assumed he couldn't hear. So we went to the specialist, we did our test, the specialist said yes, he could hear, and I was happy with that and with the fact that I too felt that he could hear. He has perfect hearing, not even a slight hearing loss.

Information on health issues associated with Down syndrome is readily available. Down syndrome association websites across the world typically include information about possible health issues, while new parent kits and information folders set out the health checks which should be undertaken as a matter of routine for a child with a disability. Yet according to the parents interviewed for this book, the level of awareness among medical practitioners about the health implications of Down syndrome and ways of dealing with people with Down syndrome, was surprisingly diverse, with parent responses to experiences with doctors and health professionals ranging from total satisfaction to incredulity and outrage. As was the case with other services, people living outside Perth sometimes found it more difficult to access the health care and information they needed and, regardless of location, parents themselves often had to be the driving force behind accessing the best service. This does not necessarily mean drawing up a battle plan. General practitioners do not always have wide experience of people with Down syndrome, but acknowledging this and being prepared to work with parents on learning about the condition can sometimes lead to a productive dialogue, as Trish Weston discovered.

If you have a baby with Down syndrome, you've actually got to educate your GP. We're very fortunate, our GP was quite frank in saying he knew nothing about Down syndrome but he's a lovely doctor and treats Will just the same as he would any of the other children and whenever I have any information about Down syndrome I pass on the information to him. Things like when I was expecting our next child and I was inquiring about having prenatal testing done, I went along to him and said I wanted a referral to go and see a specialist to talk about it. Apart from amniocentesis, he was totally unaware of any other procedures. I had to spell out to him what I wanted to know about so that he could then give me the referral to go and do that sort of stuff.

There is one area at least where doctors are in the vanguard of knowledge about Down syndrome and health — cardiology. Baby Shannon da Silva was just three months old when she had life-saving open-heart surgery in Sydney.

We learned about the need for major heart surgery pretty early on. Basically, as soon as she was strong enough to have it and before the arteries had hardened too much so that it would be impossible to perform the operation, or the operation would kill her. It wasn't presented as a choice at all. If she didn't have it, she wasn't going to survive. And as it turned out, it was enormously successful and she has a basically normally functioning heart now. There's no reason to believe that it's ever going to cause her any difficulties in the future, which is nice. (Karen Langley)

Like Shannon, Laura Middleton needed surgery as soon as she was strong enough to survive it.

Laura wasn't thriving, she was very, very skinny, a big potbelly like a kid suffering from malnutrition, and clearly wasn't doing well. The cardiologist told us she'd have to go to Melbourne for an operation, and the surgeon said she had a nineteen in twenty chance of surviving, but that's a one in twenty chance of not surviving, and that kind of shocked me a bit. And when the time came to give Laura to the nurse it was just terrible handing her over to who knows what ...

I remember coming back to the hospital after five hours and we were allowed to go down and see her in the intensive care unit pretty soon after, and there she was with fourteen tubes coming out of her, various pieces of technology attached to her, looking very small in this bed, or cot, with a kind of plastic thing over her face. She was very sick, but the nurses and the doctors in the ICU were terrific, all very encouraging. Ultimately Laura was okay to go back to the ward and after ten days or so we flew back to Perth. Then she started the process of recovery, and it seemed remarkably quick, because she started to gain all the weight she hadn't been gaining before, and got colour in her cheeks and more energy and so on. So after just two or three weeks it seemed that particular nightmare had passed and we could get on with the long run of looking after her and raising her. (Luke Middleton)

Jack Canning was a little older when he had surgery (seven months), but he hadn't experienced the same deterioration in health as had Laura.

The doctor mentioned quite early on that there could be heart problems. Jack was really healthy, he was a good size when he was born, but the paediatrician picked up a hole in his heart, quite big, and he said he would need surgery to correct that. So Jack was booked in for heart surgery at five months but just before that he had the pre-op test and they picked up a urinary tract infection. So we were all geared up and had to go home and that was really hard. And then we tried again two months later and he was fine, so we went through with it. Although it was a big hole, it was quite a simple procedure. It was just patching the one hole. It was terrible, but we were very prepared. Princess Margaret Hospital was great, they showed us pictures, told us what to expect. It wasn't shocking but it was *hard* to see him like that and in that pain but he recovered very quickly and he got over it really fast. His heart is fine now. (Britt Canning)

Britt Canning also made an observation shared by many other parents — how little the disability mattered in the face of life-threatening cardiac issues.

I remember at the time in the hospital Jack actually seemed to have quite a mild problem compared to what a lot of the kids had. And he was definitely going to recover from that heart surgery but there were kids in there who *weren't* definitely going to recover. So it helped me to put things in perspective, Jack's Down syndrome in perspective, because all I wanted was for him to get through that heart surgery and survive. So the Down syndrome was nothing then.

Living in the Kimberley the Brooktons had to wait longer than most families for a diagnosis, both of Mark's Down syndrome and then of his heart condition. As soon as the condition was picked up, the family were on a plane to Perth for immediate surgery. Not confident of a successful outcome Wendy and Keith prepared for the worst by taking photos of their baby.

It was pretty hard going. What was supposed to be one day in intensive care turned out to be ten days. He just didn't pick up. Just didn't want to breathe on his own. They removed the breathing apparatus, the breathing tube, and had to put it back in again, that was pretty hectic ...

But afterwards the difference in Mark was huge. All of a sudden, what an alive baby! Just about two weeks later he was sitting up and doing all the things he should have been doing. Had heaps more strength and colour, a big difference, yes.

Since the 1980s, open-heart surgery has become a much more routine procedure for children with congenital heart defects. Earlier, when outcomes were not nearly as promising — overall survival rates were much lower than they are today, with some evidence that children with Down syndrome experienced higher post-operative mortality[58] — there was a tendency to argue that children with Down syndrome and a heart defect had as much chance of surviving their first year without a heart operation as with one. But now, children with Down syndrome undergo surgery for congenital heart defects as routinely as anyone else, and with equally positive outcomes.[59] In Western Australia, children have been able to undergo major heart surgery in Perth since at least the early 2000s. Prior to that they were flown to Melbourne for surgery, like Laura Middleton, and even now, the most complex cases are still treated there.[60]

According to Perth paediatric cardiologist Dr Luigi D'Orsogna, who has overseen the cardiac care of a significant proportion of the state's children with Down syndrome, screening at birth for the possibility of a heart defect should be standard procedure for children with Down syndrome.

Everyone's aware of the fact now that babies with Down syndrome need to have cardiac screening. Once it was thought that it was sufficient to just listen with your stethoscope and hope to pick up a heart murmur. The recommendation now is that any baby with Down syndrome, unless they've had a foetal echocardiogram, needs to have an ultrasound done after birth, or when the condition is diagnosed. Initially it was thought that they should just have an electrocardiogram and a listen, because that was what was commonly available, but now that ultrasound echocardiography is available, that's the current recommendation that comes from the paediatric section of the Australia–New Zealand Cardiac Society. I wouldn't have thought that any doctor now would make a diagnosis of Down syndrome and then send you on your way for no further follow-up. That baby needs further assessment, because there are issues other than the heart, and also just in terms of the long-term management ...

If a child with a significant heart defect does not undergo corrective surgery the likelihood of heart failure — which means, not cessation of the heart but inadequate or incompetent functioning — is very high. Long-term outcomes could include terminal damage to the heart, the arteries and the lungs.

Children born in the twenty-first century now have heart defects corrected early, and in rural areas too, visiting cardiologists provide appropriate screening for heart issues. But cardiac specialists still see the tragic results of untreated heart defects in young adults born in the 1970s and 80s. Most are by now experiencing Eisenmenger syndrome, the end stage of heart and lung disease.

If a child with an uncorrected heart defect survives their first year, then they can go through a honeymoon period, a period of time where they become a lot better and they don't breathe as fast, they're not working as hard, they start putting on weight, and they start behaving like a child without a heart problem. They go through that period for five, ten, fifteen years. But then they become gradually bluer and bluer and they develop problems with progressive cyanosis which is the medical term for the blueness or lack of oxygen in the blood. That's a relentless process — it continues and it worsens with time and they become bluer and bluer to the point where they die from that, because they have insufficient flow going to the lungs. Usually it's a condition that will develop and be a problem by late teenage, early twenties. It's uncommon for people with Eisenmenger to live longer than thirty. (Dr Luigi D'Orsogna)

Once issues regarding the heart have been excluded or managed, parents often face more mundane problems. Respiratory tract infections for example: most parents interviewed had memories of winters of 'green noses', the situation for children with Down syndrome possibly made more difficult to manage because of their smaller facial features and nasal and ear canals. Consequently sinus and chest congestion and ear infections are a common occurrence. Many children spend most of their early winters on antibiotics, though the situation seems to improve as children get older and stronger.

Some children with Down syndrome have a slightly larger tongue than is optimal for their smaller mouths and this can lead to what is sometimes seen as a characteristic of Down syndrome, the protruding tongue. The situation can also be caused by hypotonia or lax muscle tone. As a family we attacked this issue when our daughter was very young. Every time Maddie's tongue crept out between her lips, one of her parents or her sister would say, 'Pop it in, Maddie,' and gently push it back into her mouth. It worked; and when I look at the many young people I know with Down syndrome these days, I find it hard to think of a single one who has a problem with a protruding tongue, in contrast to the stereotype.

A protruding tongue is socially unattractive, but an over-large tongue can cause breathing difficulties, as Ana Diaz discovered.

Benita had a tongue operation because her tongue was very thick and very wide, and when she got tonsils or asthma she would suffocate, because her tongue was so big. We couldn't find anyone to do the operation here. My husband wanted me to go to America, but a doctor in Sydney finally found a doctor for me here in Perth. I think she was about five years old.

Though it improved Benita's capacity to breathe normally, surgery to reduce the size of the tongue is not common. More usual is the removal of enlarged tonsils and adenoids to help prevent breathing problems and associated sleep difficulties.

When Gareth was younger, he never slept the whole night through. He's always had trouble breathing and lay with his head back and snoring and did wake himself up often to the point where at the age of eight we had his tonsils and adenoids removed, not for an infection reason, but for a sleep reason, and he has slept better since then. Well, he still does tend to sleep with his head tilted back and he snores a bit but it's nowhere near what it used to be, so I wish we'd done that earlier; but you tend not to put your children under anaesthetic if you can avoid it. (Lisa Greenwood)

Overall, respiratory conditions are now dealt with for children with Down syndrome through the use of antibiotics and the generally enhanced health routines which are available to most children living in their own homes. The days when children with Down syndrome, even with no heart defect, could still not anticipate reaching their twentieth birthday because of the likelihood of complications from a chest or respiratory infection have passed, along with the institutions where those conditions were harboured.

Gastrointestinal problems are another condition which affects people with Down syndrome disproportionately. About one in ten babies with Down syndrome have some kind of gastrointestinal abnormality, and some of these can be life threatening if not dealt with immediately. In 2008 Emily Howard's son Joe had such a condition, duodenal atresia, corrected as soon as he was born. When Amber Ravi was born in 1992 her mother Jennifer noticed there was a problem even before the nursing staff did when, forty-eight hours after her birth, Amber had still not had a bowel movement. She had an imperforate anus (the absence of a normal anal opening) which required an immediate colostomy. Repairs were not concluded till a couple of years later when a new anal opening was created surgically. Since then, Amber's parents have helped her to maintain a high fibre diet and good bowel health and habits, though she does have some continuing bowel problems and occasionally still needs enemas. Amber's experience and its resolution are fairly typical of children who have a malformation of the digestive tract.

Britt Canning's son Jack developed bowel problems when he was a little older.

He's turning eleven and he's still not going to the toilet independently. His bowel is very stretched from chronic constipation. Constipation doesn't sound like a big thing, but it can be a huge problem over many years. He wasn't a constipated baby, it started when he was four and I was trying to toilet-train him but now he's got what's called megacolon [sometimes related to Hirschsprung's disease], which is a large intestine that is very slack, there's no muscle tone, the nerves aren't working properly. So towards the end of last year he had a tube put in that connects to his appendix, which leads into his large intestine to his caecum; and we do manual washouts with a drip, at this stage about every second day, to try and wash him out so that his bowel will have a chance to shrink back to a normal size over the next several years. That's his only hope now of ever having normal bowel function. The fact that he doesn't have normal bowel function has affected his ability to go to the toilet independently so we're hoping this will work, but it's definitely going to be a very gradual process.

Conditions such as Hirschsprung's disease or an imperforate anus can make bowel training more challenging, while others which affect digestion can impact on feeding and weight gain.[61] Though inconvenient, most of these conditions are correctable or manageable.

For some reason, the incidence of leukaemia in people with Down syndrome is, at about one per cent, significantly higher than in the rest of the population.[62] For the Greenwood family the diagnosis of cancer brought back all the memories of the day when Gareth had been diagnosed with Down syndrome thirteen years previously; yet because of that earlier traumatic experience, this family seemed better prepared to deal with the new crisis. With a background in science and knowledge of the possibilities associated with Down syndrome, Lisa Greenwood was in an excellent position to overcome her shock after the family's frantic dash to Fremantle Hospital with a critically ill son, and to focus on what was important.

They gave him antibiotics and he started to calm down, and his heart rate came down a bit once they got the fluids and things into him. We were just hanging around waiting for the result of his blood test to come back. The paediatricians came down and checked him out and didn't like the look of him particularly. Then I heard two staff behind us saying, 'The white blood count's low' ... So I said to my husband Douglas, 'They're looking for leukaemia,' because I knew there's a higher risk of leukaemia in children with Down syndrome. I mean, he looked horrible; he was really, really ill. About five minutes later the paediatricians came over and they sat us down and said, 'His red blood cells have gone, he's got anaemia, which is why he's gone so pale. He has very few platelets clotting his blood. And his white cells are low which all indicate possible leukaemia.' We both just looked and said, 'Yes, so what do we do?' The nurse who was there said, 'You haven't fallen apart!' And Douglas said to them, 'Well, my wife told me five minutes ago that you were looking for leukaemia.' We sort of took it the same as we did when he was born basically. We never actually thought, 'Why us?' or all this sort of doom, gloom; it was, 'Well okay, what do we do about it? Where do we go from here?'

Though dealing with the trauma of a child with a life threatening illness such as cancer is much the same whether or not your child has Down syndrome, there are a few differences. The Greenwoods found, for example, that strategies they had developed in response to Gareth's disability proved useful in encouraging him to accept unpleasant treatments.

A week, two weeks before he got ill, was the first time I'd ever given him a tablet. I'd always syringed liquid medicine into him, painkillers and things. Two weeks before I thought, 'Oh, you're a thirteen year old, try swallowing this.' He did, he put a Panadol in his mouth and swallowed it. So now in the first weeks of treatment he's swallowing fourteen tablets at a time. Fourteen in the morning and ten at night, it's just unbelievable the number of tablets he had to swallow. He was so ill he just swallowed them, there was no arguing. But to a certain extent with Down syndrome you tend to make your children compliant, to be able to work around and get them to do what you want. That's been a benefit, in that whenever he said, 'No, I don't want to do it,' we've always said, 'Come on, you need to do this first and then we can put the TV back on,' or whatever. Now he's used to it, he's in a routine, but I saw a lot of other kids on the ward who have never had to do things. Some parents have never learnt those strategies to get their child to do something because they haven't had to before, and the parents are suffering because they can't get the child to swallow the tablets. So the advantage of having a child with Down syndrome is that we'd already learnt those strategies and techniques to get him to do what we wanted. Sounds horrible, but you know what I mean? So we can get him to have an X-ray or an MRI or whatever. Doesn't like it, tells us he's frightened, which is fine; you do what you have to do, you say, 'Yes, I know you're frightened and you're scared, but you need to do it and then we'll be able to go back to your room and do something nice.' So you've got that 'You've got to do this first and then you can do that' strategy. That's made it easier for him, and for us.

In Gareth's case too, the low muscle tone associated with Down syndrome complicated matters when he developed a serious infection in his leg. Treatment generally was also compromised because of Gareth's disability, though there may be some positive effects also, which are undoubtedly an area for further scientific research.

He ended up going from 45 kilos down to 37 kilos. He looked almost like a concentration camp survivor, compared to what he was; he certainly lost heaps of weight and muscle tone. As a result of leg surgery, and losing muscle and lying in intensive care and the fact that he's got Down syndrome anyway so his muscle tone is low, mobility became an issue. He couldn't walk at all — couldn't stand, couldn't walk. So we ended up staying in hospital for three months, then using a wheelchair for another eighteen ...

Every time he has a batch of treatment, whether it's high dose or low dose, it takes his body about four weeks to recover and get his blood cell count back up and his immunity levels up high enough for them to do the next bit, whereas a lot of people will just go from one treatment to the next, which is why they say it takes six or seven months of high dose treatment, whereas Gareth's has taken twelve months because he's had big gaps in between. And the longer those gaps are the more chance, the more people start thinking, his counts are not coming back up because it's recurring and he's relapsed. So that's always in the back of your mind, even though you don't concentrate on it ...

What we've observed, and from what they've said, the chemo does appear to hit people with Down syndrome harder. Their immunity levels drop quicker and stay down longer. But also it has a slightly better cure rate in that when it hits the bad cells, it hits the cancer cells well and truly and seems to knock them out easier too. So they do sometimes say that people with Down syndrome have a slightly greater chance of being cured completely. But that's not necessarily just Down syndrome, it's various other things as well. There are also some genes or indicators that they can pick up and if you've got them they can tell you your chances are much better. So they are starting to learn more and more about what are indicators.

Knowing how Gareth felt about his illness was hard to ascertain but Lisa was optimistic about his capacity to deal with it.

It's hard to get that indication of what he thinks because he doesn't talk and express that much of what he's going through. The thing I've noticed though from the Down syndrome side of things is that he's not suffering from depression, which I've noticed in some of the other kids in PMH [Princess Margaret Hospital]. Because they're teenagers and they're going through all their appearance type things and peer group pressures and all that sort of stuff and trying to cope with leukaemia, or cancers of any sort, and treatments and losing their hair, sometimes they're down and you can actually see it. People are very aware that they need to keep watching them. But Gareth just keeps going. He's back to his bubbly personality and nothing matters and off he goes. So that's been an advantage because we haven't had to deal with the 'Woe is me, life's horrible, I don't want to live any more.' The only indication I've got that he does know — and it's a weird indication, it's like mother's instinct — is that one of his favourite songs at the moment, which he sings really loud in the car, is one by Robbie Williams, where he sings 'I hope I'm old before I die'. Every time he bursts out, 'I like this, it's my favourite!'

Gareth has now completed high school, goes bowling with his mates, listens to music and is embarking on adult life. In 2008 he celebrated his seventeenth birthday with a massive party in a local community hall. He has an impressive scar on his leg but seems otherwise unscathed.

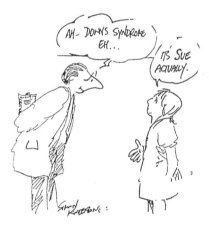

Copyright Simon Kneebone. Used with permission.

Improved health outcomes over the past decade for children such as Gareth, Amber, Shannon and Mark, measured in terms of life expectancy and quality of life, have been extraordinary, but social attitudes have not always kept up with advances in medical technology.

As the cartoon suggests, some doctors seem to see the disability of the patient before they see the patient as a person requiring treatment. Moreover they regard the parents in the same way, and they too become a focus of interrogation.

I don't say, 'Here's my Down syndrome, can you tell me what's wrong with him?' I never mention that unless it's relevant. Initially, when he was small, professional people would sort of try and find out whether I even knew that he had Down syndrome. Then if they figured out that I did know, they would launch into, 'Did you have a normal pregnancy?' Then it's open slather, and that used to irritate me and I'm quite relieved that I don't have to be constantly meeting new medical professionals and I don't have to pour out the whole history every time. (Loretta Muller)

Other doctors too were sometimes unable to get beyond their view of the parent as 'parent of a child with an intellectual disability'.

There was a doctor at our local medical practice and every time I went she would always tell me about her partner who had a daughter with an intellectual disability. This doctor would always say, 'She just can't cope with her periods and we have to sew her pads into her knickers.' Whether I had Laura with me or not, she would tell me this story! I had visions of people with intellectual disabilities throwing their pads around and this kind of stuff. What was she trying to tell me — that I should book in my toddler for an early hysterectomy? I really felt, I don't need to know this! (Jude Lawrence)

Although confident that the situation has improved since the 1980s, Trish Weston was fairly scathing about the way in which so many doctors she encountered perceived both her and her son.

It always amazed me, but I'd walk in with Will and one of the questions they would *always* ask at our first appointment was, how old was I when I had him, and the first couple of times I answered, and then after that I thought, 'I'm sorry, but is this actually relevant?' So I started earning myself the title of 'difficult parent' fairly early on. But there were things like that, and the surreptitious examining of Will's palms to see if he had a single crease, which he hasn't, so that always threw them a little bit! I guess that whole thing, that the medical profession still operates under these kind of myths — you know, older mother, single palmar crease and severe intellectual disability — it's a real worry to me.

Dealings with medical professionals transformed quite a number of people, mothers in particular, into 'difficult parents'. Many were surprised at their own assertiveness but quickly realised that in this question of their child's health, they would have to be their child's fiercest advocate. In the case of a child with a disability, parents frequently complained that the disability became an excuse proffered by some health professionals for what could otherwise be considered inadequate treatment; or else doctors declined to offer a particular service or treatment solely on the grounds of the child's disability.

In the late 1980s, Helen Golding's daughter Charlotte was experiencing difficulties with her hearing. A first attempt at inserting grommets had been unsuccessful, according to the follow-up audiology report.

I went back to the specialist with the audiology report and he then informed me that her ear canals were extremely small and that it had been a very difficult procedure and possibly the grommets were not even through the eardrum. He hadn't told me any of this at the time. So he then did an examination and decided that, 'No, they weren't in the eardrum, so we will do it again.' I made the mistake of saying to him, 'Well, is there any point in doing it again if you couldn't get it through before? I don't want her having general anaesthetic if you can't actually do the procedure. Should we be looking at maybe using hearing aids?' And he said, 'There is no point in giving her hearing aids, she is disabled' ... Then he basically threw me out of the hospital, told me not to come back if I wasn't prepared to do what he said. He wasn't impressed with me; never mind, I wasn't impressed with him either! So I walked out of the hospital thinking to myself, 'Well, that is all very good, now what do you do next? You have this child who can't hear, what are you going to do about it?' ...

What I did do was go to a Commonwealth-funded hearing facility in Fremantle which was absolutely wonderful. They did a full audiology assessment. They fitted her with hearing aids, which made a big difference and they then did a follow-up on that. We were also fortunate, if having a hearing loss is a fortunate thing to have, because once she needed hearing aids, she then qualified to use the Education Department's hearing services program. So she was able to get a preschool placement, a kindergarten placement at Mosman Park at their kindergarten.

Jude Lawrence and her daughter had a comparable experience.

Before Laura had congenital cataracts removed when she was about eighteen months old, we went to a range of specialists for second opinions. We spoke to one ophthalmologist who said that one of the options for children after that kind of surgery would be contact lenses. 'But,' he said, 'of course that wouldn't be an option in your daughter's case.' Why not? Not because she was eighteen months old, as I might have thought, but because she had Down syndrome so she wouldn't be able to cope — as if all the other eighteen month old babies would somehow cope better with contact lenses!

Although her parents ultimately decided that glasses were a better option, Laura did in fact have contact lenses for almost two years, but the family did not go back to that particular ophthalmologist.

More open-minded doctors were sometimes prepared to trust a parent's judgement. Ana Diaz wanted her daughter Benita to have braces to correct a problem with an overcrowded mouth. The orthodontist was reluctant on the grounds that perhaps Benita, with her disability, wouldn't be able to cope with the discomfort and the care routine.

But at her first follow-up the doctor said she's a model for other ones, because her teeth were so clean and so good. And she never complained.

Negative experiences with doctors are not always necessarily to do with a child's disability, but simply to do with the way some doctors relate to children. Like Helen Golding, Brenda Harvey ran foul of a hearing specialist because she dared to ask about alternatives to grommets.

I was very grateful for the hearing tests and at the Albany Hospital the audiologists there were very good, and very good with Grace, unlike a specialist I went to see, thinking that I should get a second opinion. He was totally obnoxious and really didn't know how to treat little children, let alone a Down syndrome child. He was dreadful and was so rushed that he really didn't have the time for us. He got Grace and just plonked her down on a chair, didn't say hello to her or try and get any sort of bonding happening with her, put some earphones on her and as he was walking away from her, he said, 'Say yes if you can hear anything.' And she was just a little girl at that stage, maybe four years old. And she just sort of sat there staring at him and there was no way that she would respond to that, even if she had heard a sound. There was no way she would have! So he said, 'Oh, she's deaf!' And started writing — didn't even look at me. 'She's deaf!' And I knew that he was going to suggest grommets and I said, 'Look, I've already gone through all of this. I know she has a mild hearing deficiency and I don't want her to have the grommets. I'm here to ask you, what would the problem be if you've got fluid sitting in the middle ear for a long period of time?' And he virtually told me that I was a bad mother because I wasn't going to do what he said! But before leaving, I told him how rude he was; he just outraged me enough to speak my mind to him. I then proceeded to burst into tears once I got outside of his room. So that wasn't very successful!

Some families found that living outside the metropolitan region limited their access to good health advice or services that city dwellers might take for granted. In the south-west, neither Brenda Harvey nor Loretta Muller were advised of the need to have their child's hearing and vision tested in their early years. Fortunately Loretta had been comparing notes with a friend in Canberra, whom she had met shortly after they both had children with Down syndrome. That friend had taken her son to an ophthalmologist, so Loretta decided she would take Cameron too. In fact he had quite severe astigmatism. And his father recalled how Cameron's heart murmur was also picked up by chance.

It's actually what they call an 'innocent' murmur and there is no drama with it at all and it will never get worse or anything. I think it was taking him to a GP, who listened and heard it. And then we went to a heart specialist and he did all the tests. (Andrew Danes)

These are the sorts of conditions which parents in cities are generally advised to have checked as a matter of course.

Brenda's daughter Grace did not have her sight and hearing tested until she started kindergarten, and Brenda only discovered when Grace was about seven that they had missed out on many other health checks which are advisable for children with Down syndrome. As she said, 'There's things I am realising that other children have had checked a long time ago and we haven't had any of that.' Where she had sought help it had not always been forthcoming. She once asked for her daughter's vision to be checked but the doctor 'just put a few hundreds and thousands in her hand and asked her if she could see them,' and her attempt to find out about the significance of Grace's hearing loss ended in a fight with the hearing specialist and tears. Brenda also felt her daughter might have been disadvantaged because her thyroid levels weren't tested.

> I was cross that they hadn't suggested that earlier because it could have affected her development quite a lot and she may have had that since birth. I don't know if they could have detected that earlier or not. She wasn't putting on weight. She looked all right. She was growing — height wise she was. But the weight — it wasn't in line with the height. So that went on for quite a while, and that was when they suggested to check the thyroid. So there was big changes after that.

In Western Australia, routine blood tests at birth alert doctors to conditions such a congenital hypothyroidism, but thereafter clinical assessment is important and in people with Down syndrome, thyroid imbalance is something which doctors should be quick to consider. When Trudy Fisher was put on thyroxine in 1989, her grandmother Iris was told that 'in fact she'd been a borderline for two years' but that for people with Down syndrome this was considered 'normal'. About the time Trudy's borderline thyroid function was acknowledged as a problem by her doctor, her speech pathologist had also raised the issue.

> Because her comprehension suddenly showed signs of deteriorating, and comprehension can be an early sign of thyroidism. Her comprehension suddenly started to lag behind other things, and it was very interesting to know that in fact she had been on this borderline. So at the end of April she was given thyroxine. Almost at this time, it was beginning to be realised that a lot of Down syndrome children had this thyroid problem and I was very interested in what was beginning to be talked about because I was convinced, well, this could be extremely interesting for Trudy's future academic chances. In a matter of maybe a month, two months down the track, Trudy suddenly became a chatterbox, for want of a better word. I was getting it from all regions — from the Brownies, from school, from after-school care. She really blossomed.

Tragically, Iris's granddaughter died of heart complications within months.

Sandra Rossi had surgery in Perth at the age of thirteen to correct a deformity of her femur, which had led to constant dislocation of her hips,[63] and it took her almost eighteen months to learn to walk again afterwards. From that point, back home in the Kimberley, she began to put on weight which her mother Janet thought was caused by the surgery, her daughter's continuing inability to exercise and her restricted mobility.

> It's not so much about what she eats I think because she's not a big eater; she more or less eats what we eat and I try to keep her on light stuff to help her weight problem. She

doesn't like sweets, or anything like that, so she doesn't indulge in any of those sorts of things.

Sandra also began to suffer from disrupted sleep patterns.

During the day she's out of whack, she's overtired and sleepy and stuff like that, and sometimes it gets very frustrating for her carer. This has been going on now for the last three or four years. I mean, she can't help it if she's not having a good sleep — it leaves her sort of drained and unmotivated and everything else. She gets to the stage where she's got dark circles under her eyes and she just really doesn't know whether she's coming or going.

In her twenties, increasingly overweight and with sleep problems, Sandra had never been tested for thyroid or for diabetes and had not seen a Disability Services Commission doctor. Her mother was told by the doctors she did see — 'they're regular doctors, yes; they sort of come and go' — in the Kimberley that people with Down syndrome 'didn't get thyroid problems'.

They said they've never come across a Down syndrome that had high blood pressure or high sugar. They think, well because she's a Down syndrome, that's the way it is, and there's not much you can do about it. They don't sort of take her as an individual person that has rights and needs like anybody else.

Though unhappy with the level of treatment available locally and concerned about her inability to deal with her daughter's health issues, Janet had little alternative. In any case, her experience of health care when she had accompanied Sandra to Perth for her hip operation had not made her optimistic that she could get better service for her daughter outside the Kimberley.

I was just shocked at, I suppose, the nursing attitude towards someone with a disability. They never took the time out to explain what they were doing, they just assumed that she didn't know, or they couldn't communicate with her, and they just did things without explaining. And jabbing needles and stuff like that, that was just freaking her out. Yes, she was very traumatised by it. That's when I thought there's room for improvement.

Jill Mather made the same observation of the treatment experienced in hospital by her brother Richard, a middle-aged man with Down syndrome.

It didn't matter how often we explained. Well-intentioned staff who were kind people would walk into the room and they would say to him, 'Rich, we're just going to pop in a catheter.' He said, 'Fine.' I said, 'Rich, they're going to put a tube up your penis so the wee can get out.' 'Uggh!' A slightly different proposition! 'Rich, on a scale of one to ten, how's your pain?' No ability to understand. And as a classic example, the night they brought him from ICU up to the ward, they had inserted a morphine pump and they handed him the green tab and said, 'When your pain gets too severe, press this.'

Health care is an issue for all Western Australians living outside the larger metropolitan regions but parents and carers of a person with a disability need to be particularly proactive. Even institutions such as the Aboriginal Medical Service, a boon for Aboriginal families in more remote regions like the Kimberley, had nothing available about disabilities when

Malia Lambert was born in 2002, though her mother Carol pointed out the need to them and perhaps things changed as a result. Malia had a hole in the heart which was followed up but did not require surgical intervention, but by the age of three, like children a decade earlier in Albany in the south-west, Malia had never had her eyes or ears checked. Carol herself took the initiative in following up on services such as physio, OT and speech through the LAC (local area coordinator) and the Disability Services Commission (DSC) representative in the region, who put her in contact with the Down Syndrome Association (DSA) in Perth, but it was not until she received the DSA fact file that Carol realised the need to have other health conditions checked and excluded.

A recent study of mortality of infants with Down syndrome in Western Australia in the 1980s and 90s indicated that the survival rate for Aboriginal children with Down syndrome is lower than for non-Aboriginal children, and that Aboriginal children with Down syndrome are much less likely to survive past the age of twelve years than non-Aboriginal children with Down syndrome.[64] Aboriginal children born with Down syndrome are also more likely to have a lower birth weight, which significantly impacts on their capacity to survive surgery in the event of a congenital heart defect and also indicates a reduced capacity to cope with other health complications. This is in line with the generally poorer health outlook for Aboriginal people compared with non-Aboriginal people in Australia, but factors such as distance, remoteness and differential access to education that so often distinguish the lives of Aboriginal families in areas like the Kimberley, and the growth of more widespread and pressing health issues such as foetal alcohol syndrome, suggest little immediate prospect for improvement in the circumstances of Aboriginal children with Down syndrome in regional or remote Australia.[65]

On the whole, the health outlook for people with Down syndrome in the last few decades is increasingly positive, and life expectancies are extending with every new advance and treatment. The corollary of this is that people with Down syndrome are now increasingly prone to experience the down side of a longer life span. Conditions such as being overweight or obese, the legacies of affluence and a passive lifestyle, impact as significantly on people with Down syndrome as on the rest of the population and can be managed the same way, through judicious exercise and a balanced diet and lifestyle. Mental health issues can also emerge as people age. More significant and less easily managed is the link between Down syndrome and Alzheimer's disease, with people with Down syndrome more prone to develop the changes in the brain which are characteristic of Alzheimer's disease.[66] According to studies reported on by the Alzheimer's Association of Australia, the extra 21st chromosome in people with Down syndrome means that they make one-and-a-half times as much of the damaging protein which forms plaque in the brain and seems to cause deterioration. It seems likely that all people with Down syndrome who die by the age of forty have some evidence of this type of change in the brain. But paradoxically, this does not mean that all people with Down syndrome who attain the age of forty will exhibit Alzheimer's. As Alzheimer's Australia reports, despite this finding, 'a significant number of people with Down syndrome are older than forty and show no signs of having Alzheimer's disease. It is not currently understood why changes to the brain that are typical of Alzheimer's disease do not necessarily produce the condition in people with Down syndrome.'[67]

One thing we know of Alzheimer's is, there is a great deal more to learn. The fact that people with Down syndrome experience Alzheimer's in different ways from the rest of the population might even become a focus of research that will impact beneficially on health outcomes for people with Down syndrome. In the meantime, older people with Down syndrome do experience Alzheimer's and in significant numbers. For medical practitioners, making an accurate diagnosis can be particularly problematic in the case of a person with an intellectual disability, as other conditions to which the Down syndrome population is more prone, such as thyroid, can present in ways which incorrectly suggest Alzheimer's. Further, limited communication skills, particularly among older people with Down syndrome who have not had the advantage of early educational opportunities or who have been institutionalised for long periods, combined with tests for Alzheimer's which do not take sufficient account of an existing intellectual disability, may also promote an incorrect diagnosis of Alzheimer's. For that reason, early baseline testing for Alzheimer's (which establishes a starting point for assessing change in an individual's capacity) and the involvement of family and carers in working with medical practitioners where Alzheimer's is suspected is critical.

From 2007, in response to negotiations between the Australian government, the Royal Australian College of General Practitioners and the disability sector, changes to Medicare rebates were introduced to encourage longer health checks for people with intellectual disabilities. The Disability Discrimination Commissioner Graeme Innes explained that, 'this extra rebate for General Practitioners will ensure they take the extra time needed in consultations with people with intellectual disabilities to ensure that conditions, especially the more complex ones, are checked.'[68] This initiative represents an important recognition of the health needs of people with intellectual disabilities, at all stages in their lives. Requirements include proper and timely diagnosis of medical conditions in children; non-discriminatory treatment; continuing access to quality health care which takes account of particular social and personal needs, and all offered in the context of a system which gives due recognition to the special needs of the individual and the role which family and carers can play in protecting them. As this chapter has argued, Down syndrome itself is not a medical condition, but it can lead to negative health outcomes. In the twenty-first century however, caring and inclusive health care is bringing about increasingly positive outcomes.

In 1998, stimulated by concern about the standard of health care routinely made available to people with Down syndrome, the Down's Syndrome Association in the United Kingdom surveyed its membership about their experiences. The subsequent report was entitled tellingly, 'He'll never join the army'. Of 1509 responses, 72 per cent were satisfied with the level of care they had received, but 28 per cent (426 respondents) were not, a finding which came on the heels of what had supposedly been 'a decade of commitment to the health care of people with disabilities' in the United Kingdom, embodied in two Department of Health reports, which leaves one wondering what the level of dissatisfaction might have been ten years earlier.[69] It takes a survey of that magnitude to really dredge the depths of the 'medical horror stories' many people with Down syndrome and their families have filed away. In Western Australia, the horror stories are certainly there, but there seems to be less evidence of the entrenched denial of the right to decent health care which many British families — more than one quarter — evidently had to contend with. Undoubtedly a greater knowledge of Down syndrome within the general medical profession as a whole would be desirable. So too would be wider provision of medical services in the regions, which remains an issue for Western Australians whether or not they have a disability.

In matters such as access to life-saving cardiac surgery, ICU and hospital care, all the Western Australian families I spoke to seemed extremely happy with the excellent standard of medical care their family members received as a matter of course. The attitude which led to the death of Christopher Derkacz in Princess Margaret Hospital in 1979 is seemingly long laid to rest, at least within intensive care units. But this is not necessarily enough. Many of the everyday conflicts with doctors described in this chapter may seem minor, even amusing; but medical attitudes are also shaped by, and are intrinsic to, attitudes which in some cases can promote a view of people with disabilities as not worthy of the same level of care as others, and by implication, not quite good enough to participate fully in our society. The problem is not necessarily one for the people who are outraged and who move on or become 'difficult parents'; the problem is for those who don't realise such treatment is discriminatory and potentially damaging or even life threatening. Everyone engaged in disability and health care needs to be vigilant in acknowledging the right of people with disabilities to excellent health care, and to reject anything which smacks of second best.

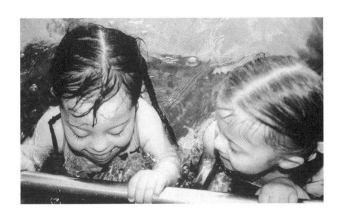

chapter 4

GIVING HOPE A HELPING HAND

Having accepted that they are taking a child with a disability into their homes, for most parents the question that follows 'Why?' and 'Why us?' is, 'What on earth are we going to do now?' Parents have always responded to this in terms of the historical context of disability. In the 1940s and 50s few if any services were available for children with intellectual disabilities, deemed to be ineducable and untrainable and their unfortunate condition beyond intervention, and on that basis little was expected of parents who chose to keep their children at home beyond keeping the child fed and clothed and perhaps loved until its likely early demise. Increasingly however, parents and professionals began to challenge this fatalism. Partly through their efforts and partly because of the impact of radical worldwide changes to the conceptualisation of people with intellectual disabilities, services and support have emerged which most parents nowadays are able to take for granted.

Perhaps we also take for granted the meaning behind the availability of services. When our daughter was born in 1992, and we learned that Down syndrome meant not just an intellectual disability but delayed physical development, one of our first questions to our paediatrician was, what about trying things like physiotherapy? His response was that we would hear a lot about what 'these kids' could achieve, and maybe physiotherapy might get them there a little faster, but ultimately, they would go as far as they were going to go and no further: so why bother? We accepted his advice uncritically and stoically — we had feared the situation was useless — but within days we learned with astonishment not only that a whole range of therapies was available under the rubric of early intervention, but that kids with Down syndrome were talking, reading and writing, swimming, dancing and doing gym, playing judo, netball, scrabble and musical instruments, graduating from high school ...

Surely, we reasoned, if services were provided as a matter of course, and if everyday kids with Down syndrome were thriving, seemingly as a consequence of encouragement and faith, that must mean there was hope? Suddenly a life term with no remission had been commuted to a suspended sentence. Our paediatrician's ill-informed words represented the mindset of the 1950s; the availability of services and the concrete evidence we saw of what people with Down syndrome could achieve if just given the necessary support, revived the hope our paediatrician had sought so misguidedly to kill off. We immediately decorated Maddie's hospital crib with brightly coloured pictures and installed a transistor radio, to kick-start the process of stimulation.

The existence of realistic positive expectations for the future of their children, and concrete pathways to follow in achieving them, is surely the biggest difference between today's parents of a child with Down syndrome and those of earlier generations, as Mavis Simpson recognised. She was one of the trailblazers of the 1940s and 50s who refused to see her son institutionalised.

> I feel — and this is where the new parents have an advantage — we had very low expectations, you know, we didn't know any better at that time. It's only by our own experience that we learnt that they could be capable of a lot more, but by that time it was too late.

With their condition usually identified within a few hours of birth, babies with Down syndrome have the largest window of opportunity for accessing early intervention services, and arguably the most to gain. For some families, the need for disability-specific information, support and services once their child is born is overwhelming, though others felt that they wanted time initially to focus on their child as a newborn baby rather than a disability package. Ironically, this is not always easy. Nowadays a baby born with Down syndrome is not 'just' a baby. In Western Australia, the birth of a child with Down syndrome sets off a chain of events outside the control of parents, involving notification and the external provision of services and support. Some parents welcome the flood of intervention while others occasionally feel swamped by this wave of professional input. Those who received few services, which was the norm for families before the 1980s and can still be the case in regional Western Australia, certainly felt they could have done with more. This chapter looks at the development of government agencies such as today's Disability Services Commission (DSC) and parent groups such as the Slow Learning Children's Group and in particular the Down Syndrome Association of Western Australia (DSAWA),[70] and at the impact of the availability of support and services on the families of young children with Down syndrome.

The first wave of groups advocating on behalf of children with intellectual disabilities kept at home emerged in Australia after the Second World War. It was part of a larger international movement, which, over the second half of the twentieth century, transformed western attitudes to intellectual disability. In the 1950s some parents in Western Australia, rather than sending their children to an institution like Claremont Hospital for the Insane, chose to keep children at home, but in doing so they encountered enormous obstacles to giving them anything approaching a 'normal' life. Access to educational facilities was basically non-existent and social acceptance no better. Concerned parents gradually found one another and a discussion group which formed in the early 1950s became the Slow Learning Children's Group (SLCG),[71] its name still redolent of the times.

The aim of the SLCG was, first and foremost, to establish educational opportunities, but early goals also included setting up clinics to examine their children and to determine the nature of their longer term needs and, again looking long term, establishing respite services, holiday homes, useful work opportunities and farm colonies where young adults with intellectual disabilities could live safely and securely, independently of their families. In this, the SLCG was more ambitious than counterparts developing concurrently in the eastern states. By 1953, the SLCG had established five preschools across Perth and its own assessment clinic, Irrabeena; in 1954 it set up its own farm colony at Hawkevale.[72] Today the SLCG has become Activ Foundation, the largest provider of services to people with disabilities in Western Australia, continuing the SLCG's original focus on employment, accommodation, family support and respite, and the whole-of-life needs of people with disabilities.[73] Providing safe accommodation and continuing occupation for one's children still remains fundamental to the concerns of parents, and is discussed in later chapters.

When Trevor Simpson was born in 1943, his mother Mavis joined other parents in seeking information and services. In her case, finding a dearth of acceptable support, she set about providing it for herself and for others.

There was no support for the family really — there was nothing at all then that we were aware of. The first idea we had of any possible help was when we read in the paper that an organisation for mentally retarded children was being discussed. We went to the first meeting and that's where we caught up with a group which had been formed by parents whose children were in government schools and were, well, more or less left out, and the parents were looking to get something organised ...

Probably the first thing that was available was a centre at the Kings Park Tennis Pavilion where the Crippled Children's Society had set up a little day centre. They accepted some mentally handicapped children too, but they weren't really interested in them, because they were interested in the physically handicapped. Trevor was about six I think, when he started to go there, and he went for about a year. Transport was provided by volunteers and a cousin of mine was one of the transport drivers. I used to travel with her and it was quite difficult, really, coping with these children in a car. However, we learnt quite a bit at the centre and at least he was getting some experience of mixing with other people.

But when they decided to set up a proper association for children with physical handicaps, it was the Spastic Welfare

Association that was formed and of course the children who were not regarded as spastic were not acceptable.

In his work on parent associations and their development in Australia, Charlie Fox points to the embryonic postwar notion of the rights of children with a disability, their rights as citizens — perhaps surprisingly, in view of the contemporary understanding of the rights-based model as being the product of the 1980s and of international movements and events such as the United Nations' 1981 International Year of Disabled Persons. However, the rhetoric of rights permeated the work of University of Queensland special education professor Fred Schonell in the 1950s and 60s, and thus it was the Queensland parents' organisation, with Schonell at its head and imbued with his philosophy, that became the driving ideological force behind the parent movement.[74] The idea of a 'normal' home upbringing was already starting to emerge within these parents groups, some twenty years before Wolf Wolfensberger's normalisation model gained general acceptance, but at this stage, in the 1950s and early 1960s, institutionalising children who had diagnosed intellectual disabilities such as Down syndrome was still very much the norm. As Fox points out too, 'Doing something about the institutions themselves was not in [the parents'] aims. They felt no kin with either the disabled children in the institutions or with the parents who had put them there.'[75] In fairness, parents undoubtedly had more than enough battles to fight on behalf of their own children.

Other ideas in currency in the postwar era also facilitated shifts in understandings about disability. In the context of an emergent welfare state and the growth in the belief of betterment for all following the austerity of the war years, people with disabilities, and their families, found a place. The culture of self-help and mutual aid which was fundamental to these sorts of parent organisations was not new, although it was given new force under the Commonwealth government of Robert Menzies. But in the postwar years, as women in particular started to become more politicised within their traditional roles, the mothers of children with disabilities became increasingly vocal and largely formed the backbone of parent organisations. At the time of the formation of the SLCG, the majority of those involved were the parents of children with Down syndrome — the 'Mongoloids'.[76]

The arrival of the SLCG certainly improved things but the crucial step in the development of services for people with intellectual disability in Western Australia was the establishment in 1964 of the Mental Deficiency Division (MDD) of the state's Mental Health Services. For the first time the administration of intellectual disability was separated from the administration of mental illness, and the state accepted responsibility for the provision of services. The SLCG assessment clinic Irrabeena was absorbed into the MDD, and the name Irrabeena was later applied informally to the Authority for Intellectually Handicapped Persons (AIH), forerunner to the Disability Services Commission (DSC).[77] However, state responsibility for services did not mean all needs could be met. William Mann, recalling the family's experiences after Geoffrey was born in 1967, was adamant that 'We got no help whatever. This was one of the things that made us cranky with the system.' His wife Muriel concurred, but was more positive about how things worked out.

We were referred to Irrabeena and we heard comforting words from Dr Hamilton that he gave to everybody in those days, that in a crisis they'd help us and no intellectually handicapped person would sleep rough; they might not be in the right place, but they'd be somewhere. Well, we learnt the hard way too, that that isn't true. But at that time, I suppose, it was reasonably comforting to know that there was a backstop there.

Over this period the services offered by Irrabeena and its successors were increasingly influenced by ideas gaining currency internationally: deinstitutionalisation, normalisation and social role valorisation (SRV).[78] Normalisation, the doctrine which required that people with intellectual disability lead as normal a life as possible, arrived in Western Australia in the 1970s, to be replaced in the mid 1980s with the reworked doctrine of SRV, the term coined by American normalisation guru Wolf Wolfensberger in 1983. SRV required that people with intellectual disabilities be given roles that would be socially valued, thus facilitating their social inclusion. Importantly these doctrines or practices advocated that people with intellectual disabilities leave institutions. In 1966 dozens of children were moved out of Claremont to Pyrton Training Centre, established with a view to training its residents in living skills towards the ultimate goal of living in the community. With Claremont no longer taking children, the expectation grew that children with intellectual disabilities would be brought up with their families. As a consequence, government services were increasingly provided to children in their own homes or in the community, a pattern which was to remain in place for decades.[79]

In those early days, services often came by good luck rather than as a matter of right, and parent initiative and word of mouth would remain important.

In the late 1960s, support from Irrabeena came in. Never officially, just the occasional contact, personally or this member of the staff or that. For instance, I learnt from a neighbour that there was a patterning program at

Irrabeena to teach handicapped babies to crawl properly, and so I asked if I could bring Geoffrey along because he was very slow to learn to crawl. They wouldn't though. Down syndrome babies are always slow to crawl, so I got no help. But my friend who was working as a volunteer assisting with the patterning exercises at Irrabeena came and showed my daughters and I how to do these exercises, and then told the physiotherapist that she had done that, so the Irrabeena physiotherapist who only lived two blocks away came charging round one Saturday morning to make sure we were doing it properly! (Muriel Mann)

Apart from education and health checks, parents wanted therapies — physio, occupational (OT) and speech; but they also wanted information. While therapies were increasingly offered through Irrabeena, other elements of support weren't always available. A second wave of parent groups evolved, tied more specifically to the needs associated with particular disabilities, as parents became more assertive about exactly what they wanted, which included companionship and disability-specific information. By the mid 1980s, Down syndrome–oriented groups had begun to emerge in other states and soon there was a push for something similar in Western Australia. Many new parents were already involved in groups such as the Noah's Ark Toy Library in Perth, or attended therapy sessions or more socially oriented playgroups at Irrabeena, and a number of new and recent mothers began to organise informal coffee mornings to share their experiences. DSAWA did not grow out of dissatisfaction with government services but was more an acknowledgement of the need for peer support among parents of newborn children with Down syndrome. Trish Weston for example was delighted that her son Will, born in 1984, was getting home visits from therapists and social trainers at least every couple of weeks as part of Irrabeena's early intervention program, but recognised in retrospect that she needed something else.

> I began to see that it meant that we were quite isolated. Occasionally they would have a group session, but that wasn't happening very much at that stage. So that while we were getting individual one-to-one attention, I would have sacrificed some of that for contact in a group.

Trish had already sought out personal support when her baby was first born, visiting SLCG's family support services in the hope of finding some group contact.

> I went in there thinking that perhaps I'd be put in touch with another family or maybe they could give me some information and I sort of came away feeling like I'd been patted on the head and told that I was doing a great job and if you're going to have a baby with a disability, this is the one to have and oh, a bit patronised I suppose. I certainly didn't get what I was looking for, whatever that was, and I'm not sure I really knew what that was at that stage ...

Even where group contact was available, however, Trish and others like her found it didn't go far enough.

> Irrabeena's services were for all children in a certain age range, so it wasn't specific to Down syndrome. I mean, I would go along to those sorts of things, but the only thing I thought I had in common with other mothers was that we were getting our services through Irrabeena. But as soon as I started talking to another mum with a child with Down syndrome there *was* that bond that they understood. They knew they could share information with

me and I could do the same. Just sharing things, little helpful things like, how did you get him to sit up? Or some of the kids had legs that splayed a lot and people would share ways of keeping them together. Oh, there was lots of stuff like that.

The common bond went well beyond the practical to include a profound and sometimes almost unrecognised need for personal support.

A lot of it was just, 'Oh, I felt like this, and when this happened I felt like that,' and everyone would say, 'Oh, yes, I know! This is what happened to us too,' and I think *that* was the really important thing, that you really could cast off some of the guilt about how you felt. We would talk quite frankly about how some of the parents — probably most of us — at some stage in those early days, weeks, thought, 'If he died in his sleep it would probably be easier for everyone' — and then felt *horrible* for thinking that, for allowing that thought to even enter your mind. And when people got to actually talking we found that just about everyone had had thoughts like that, that they felt terribly guilty about. Just talking about those sorts of things establishes such a deep bond between people, and it frees you up a lot, to think that your thoughts were actually quite normal, quite natural and you shouldn't carry it around with you for the rest of your days, feeling awful about it.

Encouraged by clinic sisters who were able, sometimes clandestinely, to put them in touch with other mothers of children with Down syndrome, a few women started getting together. Jackie Softly, Christine Cooper, Maria Crawford, Christine Goodger, Ann Hardie, Lyn Parker and Marcia Rowlands were among them.[80] This was in 1985.

We used to meet in each other's homes, I think every couple of weeks, and that was wonderful. There were about half a dozen of us who used to go every single time and a few others that came in occasionally. And that was really what we needed at the time. We were all much of a similar age and we all had little babies with Down syndrome. Then someone mentioned that there was a national association in the throes of being set up and so we thought we would hold a public meeting at Noah's Ark Toy Library in North Perth to see if there was any interest in having a group in Western Australia, and we got lots and lots of people there the first time. (Trish Weston)

Ed Price, an older man with a granddaughter with Down syndrome and experience in management, had a firm belief in the need to do it 'properly' along constitutional lines and with a committee in place. From the outset he and his wife Olive were eager to be part of the proposed Down syndrome group and thirty years later, Olive Price remained a strong and active supporter of the organisation. Ed played a driving role in the early days.

There was a very simple meeting one night at someone's house and Ed sort of nominated us. 'You look like a good secretary, Jackie! And you can chair the meeting, Marcia, and Lyn can do the treasurer!' I mean, that's what it was like! He told us what to do really, pushed us into doing everything, which was probably good. (Diana Foster)

The Downs (later Down) Syndrome Association of Western Australia Inc. (DSAWA) was incorporated on 30 December 1986. At first the Association's home was Jackie Softly's dining room table, but by 1991 DSAWA had found Activ-owned premises in Churchill Avenue, Subiaco. In November the following year it had moved to an office at Meerilinga, on Hay Street, West Perth, where it stayed until 1999. For a while the Association was homeless and operated out of Cathy Donovan's living room. That was followed by a short-term shift to East Victoria Park, then another in November 2000 to Bentley, then in 2010 to South Perth. Along the way, and funded by parent membership fees, fundraising activities, donations and grants for particular projects, the Association acquired a voluntary board of management, a small paid staff (supported by volunteers) and a library of resources.

As the children of the first members have grown up, the interests of the Association have correspondingly matured, so that now the whole-life spectrum from birth to adulthood is a focus of the Association's activities. It has developed from an informal kitchen-table structure to a professionally run organisation. Publicity and advocacy for disability-specific areas are key parts of its platform and it has engaged in a number of political campaigns including support for national health initiatives for people with Down syndrome; promoting research into links between Down syndrome and Alzheimer's disease, and making major submissions to government inquiries on subjects ranging from sterilisation and social justice in the early 1990s, to education and, in 2009, disability and migration.

While DSAWA does not generally offer 'services' in the sense of therapies, it sometimes runs playgroup type activities for younger kids, and new parent mornings which provide an important venue for local networking and sometimes a source of lifelong friendships among children and parents. The Association facilitates social activities for other age groups and is a major provider of education seminars for parents, teachers, health professionals, carers and support workers through its training and consultancy team. Its trained hospital visiting team, on request, provides support visits, contact and information to new parents across the state. Communication with parents and raising public awareness about people with Down syndrome remain important activities.[81]

Though in many ways DSAWA has moved miles from its starting point, it continues to fulfil its original brief of providing support to people with Down syndrome and their families with a view to empowering individuals to achieve the best possible life for people with Down syndrome. This is done in tandem with the provision of concrete services and therapies through DSC.

As soon as their child is born parents typically want information, and the quest usually starts in hospital or with the attending doctor. Here the context, the way advice is passed on, and the parents' level of anxiety are all critical in determining how information is received and interpreted. Some parents, for example, are outraged when told 'not to worry' about the disability, whereas others, like Pamela Franklin, whose daughter Catherine was born in 1984, find the advice helpful.

A lot of women I have spoken to have had pretty grizzly experiences with doctors. But this fellow said, 'She will be all right, she's healthy.' She didn't have a heart problem, didn't have any of the other problems, and he said, 'Just take her home and treat her like you would any of your other kids.' That might not have been perfect advice but it was good at the time, because it wasn't as though he was saying, you are going to have a terrible time, she won't be able to do this, that and the other; he didn't give me any indication of what she could or couldn't do, just, 'Go home and look after her, just like you would anyone else.'

Importantly, this advice came coupled with reassurances about Catherine's health. It was also Pamela's fourth child. Trish Weston may have had less confidence about how to treat her firstborn child 'normally' and in her particular circumstances found the advice she was given, also in 1984, unhelpful.

> I wasn't given any information at all, basically. The questions that we asked were met with, 'Oh, don't worry about it,' you know, 'Just take him home and love him.' The old classic line. I knew that it was important that we should start with some sort of early intervention. I didn't know it was called that at the time, and I asked the paediatrician about that and her response was, 'Well look, if it were me I would just take him home and enjoy him as a normal baby for twelve months and then worry about it!' And that didn't suit us, so I started on a bit of a crusade to find information and help.

Trish and her husband weren't referred to Irrabeena for any services at all until, having commenced her own research into early intervention, she demanded a referral from her paediatrician. A decade later in a much more information-rich environment, first time mother Karen Langley decided that learning to parent a baby with Down syndrome would come second to simply parenting. Her daughter was born at a Canberra birthing centre in 1994.

> The midwives said, 'You have a baby who is different, but this baby is still a baby. What she needs more than anything else is for you to take her home and feed her and love her and, you know, do all the things that you do with babies,' and I think we really took that to heart and thought, okay, well, stuff this Down syndrome. We will take her home and do all of that, and that's what we did.

Karen and her husband Paolo da Silva were able to make that decision having already been offered a contact with the local Down syndrome organisation and being well down the path to accessing early intervention services. Nowadays, it's hard to imagine any parent of a child with Down syndrome born in metropolitan Western Australia being dismissed the way Trish was, without any referral to services.

In Western Australia, when a child with a disability is born, the hospital or midwife is likely to send notification to the Birth Defects Registry, a statistical register collated by Perth's largest maternity hospital King Edward Memorial Hospital and based on reports from both statutory and voluntary sources: midwives' notification systems; death certificates and hospital morbidity statistics; general practitioners and maternity hospitals.[82] These statistics have been collected since 1980 and notification was voluntary until 2009, when the state government moved to introduce statutory notification of birth anomalies.[83] There is some evidence of under-reporting of 'birth defects' among Aboriginal communities and in regional Western Australia, but the register is nonetheless thought to be fairly comprehensive.[84] Conditions recorded included chromosomal abnormalities such as Down syndrome, but also physical conditions such as cleft palate, illnesses such as cystic fibrosis, and a myriad other anomalies, such as undescended testes. Data is collated anonymously. More importantly, metropolitan hospitals also generally offer parents of a newborn child with a disability such as Down syndrome a visit from a social worker and a referral form to Disability Services. Once the form is completed, and with the child's disability confirmed by means of the cytogenetic report (blood analysis), the child and the family are eligible for disability support. The family is then referred to the local area coordinator (LAC), who guides them regarding the services available, what is appropriate for their child and how to access them.

Services generally include speech and language therapy designed to stimulate language connections as well as facilitate clear speech; physio and occupational therapy. As a child ages, other services such as podiatry become available as needed. These services, which come in tandem with health checks and referrals, are offered as part of 'early intervention', designed to give children with disabilities a developmental kick-start, and they usually phase out as a child reaches particular milestones. At different times over the years since the state first took on responsibility for providing these sorts of therapies, families have had services delivered to their homes, have travelled to centres to access them or have been funded to seek them privately.

The Manns found services less than adequate in the 1970s but in that decade provision of services was increasingly redefined by the recognition that people with intellectual disabilities could develop social and life skills if supported or trained appropriately.[85] The earlier this started the better. By the 1980s and 90s people with young children were astonished and delighted to find that services such as physiotherapy and speech therapy arrived right on their doorstep. Britt Canning's son Jack was born in 1995 and Richard Gregson's son Jordan the following year.

I had had no idea these services existed, let alone that I didn't have to pay for them, except for our taxes of course. And they came to my home, which is fantastic. I wanted to do whatever we could do to stimulate Jack and help him reach his potential from the very, very beginning, so I just felt enormously grateful. (Britt Canning)

We had no problem with therapists coming to our home. In fact we were delighted that in this modern day and age we got a very good service that comes to people, rather than people having to track down and go to them. (Richard Gregson)

While devouring all the services on offer through DSC and its predecessors Irrabeena and AIH, parents continued to pursue more individual therapy interests. In the 1980s, for example, parents from DSAWA got involved in a number of different therapy and educational activities. TRIP, transactional intervention programs, was one. The program involved parents in active intervention through play with the child, letting the child lead the play but without being too directive. Diana Foster, who 'loved it', said the approach developed from observing children and parents playing.

Most people with children with disability tend to direct their child's play, as opposed to regular children where they don't direct as much. So it's learning not to tell your child what to do, to take away their self-esteem, or to give them the power so that they had some control over their environment and learning.

Others such as the Fishers and later Luke Middleton and Jude Lawrence independently took up direct instruction programs for the development of speech, language and other cognitive skills, through organisations such as Parents as Educational Partners, and through psychologist David Leach at Murdoch University. A number, including Pamela Franklin in 1985, adopted the Doman Delacato patterning program, with Pamela organising a troop of volunteers to come to her home to assist with the intensive interaction required in this approach. This method was developed in the late 1950s specifically for use with brain-injured children but it had also been taken up for children with disabilities such as Down syndrome. Pamela was already accessing Irrabeena's services when she came across the approach.

> I had read about this Doman Delacato method and I thought that sounded like a good idea but I didn't think I would do anything official because really, you couldn't relax. You just have to keep going. But I did organise a group of people, probably about twenty people, who came in every day for an hour each pair, and just helped her rolling over. She might have been about four or five months old by then. I organised this thing where they came in between about nine o'clock and one, maybe even later, maybe the last person might have left at two. Irrabeena set up the program and I got the people.

Around the same time, Trish Weston was working with her son on a similar type of intensive therapy program facilitated by Melbourne-based Ian Hunter.

> I think Will was about ten or eleven months old and he really wasn't doing very much. He could roll over and he could sit up but he couldn't pull himself to stand and he couldn't crawl. He would get around by rolling around the place. Within a couple of weeks of starting this really intensive therapy program, he'd managed to pull himself up to stand and he was getting up onto his knees anyway, so we continued with that right up until he'd turned two. We had to get volunteers in to help him do the program for something like three or four hours a day.

In the mid 1990s Richard and Beth Gregson also set up an intensive physical therapy program, with volunteer workers coming into their house three times a week to work with their son.

Parents would focus on different activities and therapies according to their understanding of their child's individual needs and indeed their own family's interests. Early reading for example. With increased awareness over the last few decades of the capacity of children with Down syndrome for early literacy because of the groundbreaking work undertaken by Sue Buckley of Down Syndrome Education International in the United Kingdom, a number of parents in the 1990s, including Penny Innes, Karen Langley, Luke Middleton and Jude Lawrence, focused on developing reading skills in their preschool children. Even prior to this, in the days when it was assumed that kids with Down syndrome 'didn't' read, the Mann family's personal commitment to Geoffrey's literacy produced great results, as William recognised. There was no question about it for this family.

> Muriel had spent a lot of time and effort to get him to recognise words. A tremendous amount of effort she put into him. Our household was an intellectually oriented household and our expectation was that Geoffrey was going to read!

Regrettably, Geoffrey's reading skills have fallen away somewhat since joining the workforce and living independently. This is not unusual as people with Down syndrome get older, but it does reinforce the need to work on maintaining skills.

Occupational therapy for the development of fine motor skills was critical in early school years as children worked on handwriting and keyboard skills. Physiotherapy services though were generally withdrawn once children were on their feet and developing what physios like to call 'a nice gait'. Nevertheless, many families continued to find 'therapeutic' activities to enhance their children's gross motor development. Luke Middleton spoke about their success in this area.

I think the most important thing for Laura's physical development was Unigym, which was the program at the University of Western Australia run by Kerry Smith, where she went every Saturday morning. That just did so much for her. It's a physical program which is to do with ball skills, running, swimming, skipping, jumping, all those kind of skills that kids should have and sometimes don't. It was actually a course run for the human movement students and it would be their coursework to teach the kids physical skills. We had a range of really good teachers, they were terrific. She just learnt so much. The thing with kids with Down syndrome is that you have to break everything down to little bits and get kids to learn doing a particular thing in its broken-down bits, and then put them all together to do a whole activity. They would do that with all those skills that I was talking about. So when Laura first started, one of the things she had to do was run twenty-five or fifty metres in a straight line. She would zigzag up the line — it was really funny to watch actually, but after a while she was running straight up the middle of the line to the end. We kept her there longer than we should have because we could hardly bear to leave the place.

One of the areas where parents sought most help was speech, and here results were mixed. While most parents believed their children had reasonable to excellent receptive language, many regretted that their expressive language, their capacity to speak clearly or fluently, was not well developed. Further, despite intensive speech therapy, some children with Down syndrome do not become verbal, though this is the minority. While speech therapy can undoubtedly help, speech impediments and some lack of clarity in speech are fairly common among people with Down syndrome. An unfortunate outcome of this is that other people can mistakenly underestimate the comprehension of people with Down syndrome because of the challenges they face in expressing themselves clearly. Speech was the most fraught area for families and many continued with private speech therapy after DSC services were withdrawn.

Just as women were instrumental in the development of the early parent support groups, mothers rather than fathers usually took on the primary role in accessing services and implementing therapies. Pamela Franklin took this for granted in the context of her family life at the time.

> David was working and got on with it. And I was the driving force about all the things we have done for Catherine. I would discuss them with David, but there was nothing that he objected to anyway. He basically left that all to me, and he always has. He is happy for me to make the decisions in the home and I suppose that if I wasn't working, I may as well do that. There is no reason to worry him about it if I could handle it myself.

Claudia Mansour reached a similar conclusion, but in retrospect she regretted that she had not shared more information with her husband.

> He was in business and he worked at one stage seven days a week and he had great responsibilities and I thought *he* can't do it. *I* can do it. But he never accepted Theresa's condition, he never wanted to discuss it with anybody. No, not at all. When she went to those programs and I'd say to him, 'Now, when you play with her, you've got to do this, there is a special way, you have to stimulate her, you can't

just play,' he would say, 'Don't say that, there's nothing wrong with her.' It was just a total rejection of the truth, he couldn't accept. It took him years. Yes, my greatest mistake was, from day one when I went to research, we should have done it together.

Not all households are organised along traditionally gendered lines of course. Richard Gregson worked from home, so had a lot of contact with therapists visiting Jordan; Luke Middleton was lucky enough to be on long service leave in 1992, the year his daughter was born, and played a major part in attending therapy sessions, workshops and DSAWA coffee mornings, but his was not a typical role for fathers during a child's early years.

I was hanging out with the mums mostly. I didn't meet many fathers, not many went to the playgroups because they were during the day and I guess they were all working, but I've met quite a few since then.

One parent's lack of involvement in therapies though could certainly undermine their efficacy. This was evident, for example, with those families who chose to use Makaton sign language with their child. Signing is a strategy favoured by some speech pathologists as a bridge before speech emerges; a way of enhancing communication channels for children whose speech is delayed. It is not promoted universally for children with Down syndrome, however, and there is often reluctance on the part of parents to introduce it; they want their children to take their place in a speaking community and regard signing as a way of avoiding the need to speak.

We chose not to use Makaton because we have always felt, rightly or wrongly, that giving them an alternative to speech will mean that they don't *have* to learn to speak as soon. (Helen Golding)

Those who did use signing though were generally extremely enthusiastic. Lucas Tanaka was the classic textbook case. His mother Mary explained that as his speech developed, the signs dropped away. His elder brother Kenji also became involved in the process of learning and communicating with sign, which would have reinforced the benefits.

> I can tell you signing's the best thing that ever happened to Lucas. It made sense to me to sign because he wasn't communicating, so he needed somehow to communicate and he was just picking it up so well. He must have been signing from about two and a half years to four, which was a bit over a year and a half. We had a speech therapist coming three times a week. And within a year, he'd learnt how to sign and then he was speaking so well, he gave up his signing ...

> And Kenji was like a translator; he was at the sessions all the time and he'd be helping, especially for Lucas to learn to take turns, Kenji would be there and he'd be taking turns. The therapist just learnt to include him so he knew all the signs. It was really good.

Karen Langley was equally committed to signing. The family lived in Brazil for extended periods, and her daughter picked up Portuguese with minimal difficulty. Theirs is a bilingual household and Karen is adamant that signing was a deciding factor in Shannon's language ability and the fact that she took on and acquired two languages.

And, also, I think it was a major factor in getting over a lot of early frustrations, because she was able to communicate even though she couldn't speak.

But while Makaton definitely provided a bridge for some children, it still raised issues in other families, even where it was used successfully.

I really feel, to integrate and to be a part of society, he is going to need to talk. He needs to be able to communicate to get on in the world somehow and unfortunately the rest of the world doesn't know Makaton signing. (Britt Canning)

Teachers of Makaton stress that signing needs to be used as part of a daily routine. In the family situation, its use was likely to be confined to the primary caregiver and attendant at workshops (often the mother) and the child itself. The difficulties fathers often faced in picking up the approach on a casual basis often sparked the recognition that signing had some limitations.

Speech is not the only area where household gender divisions can be a problem and with this in mind, Brenda Harvey suggested that a family-oriented or even community-oriented approach was necessary to make therapies worthwhile.

With the therapists' appointments and workshops that I have been to, my husband Anil didn't go, so I have felt that it was just me getting all this information and really, for any constructive changes or happenings to be going on in the home, the whole family needs to be getting it as well. Same with the speech therapy. I was given lots of information and for me alone to be doing that, I can't see the point. I feel that the other children and Anil, all of us, and other friends, all need to be doing it as well. So, you know, that might have had a lot to do with me not taking a lot of it up, because it was actually beyond me to just do it by myself. And that must happen a lot if the men are out working. You can't come home laden up with all this information and impart it to your partner properly.

Ultimately though, while there may have been some tensions about the best mode of delivering services to maximise effectiveness, everyone who used services agreed they would have been happy to have more.

Outside Perth, the issues regarding availability and delivery of services and support can be entirely different. The process of notification and subsequent follow up or referral is much more loosely structured than in the metropolitan area. Local area coordination developed in regional Western Australia in the late 1980s and was subsequently introduced into the Perth metropolitan area as a means of effective disability service provision at a local level by drawing on existing providers and localising the distribution of services.[86] One LAC from a regional WA town described the process.

Local area coordination is all about getting to know people with disabilities and their families, helping to identify their needs to be able to stay part of the community, so that they don't have to go off anywhere else; and then working towards getting those needs met locally. So apart from working with the individual and the family, it's also about working with the community, more on the community development line of things, so the community can be responsive to the needs of people with disabilities. This is their home and this is where they can stay, getting their needs responded to. It's also about providing information to families, support and advocacy.[87]

As with the likely under-representation of disabilities among those recorded on the Birth Defects Registry for regional and Indigenous populations, there is a very high probability of under-representation on the books of regional LACs, with methods of accessing clients sometimes haphazard.

It's either through referral from a doctor, or there might be a neighbourhood house or Centrelink or whoever; they might refer the individual just to come in and see me, or people just come in through the door. Sometimes I see people down the street, and say, 'Oh did you know about us?' So any kind of way really. Family members. Often a lot of my referrals come through other agencies, who just send people over to help them out.[88]

Carol Lambert may have missed out on LAC follow-up and referral to services because when her daughter Malia, born in 2002, was still young, she and her family moved from one part of the huge Kimberley region to another, the family taking up residence on a fairly isolated Aboriginal community with just one telephone line, miles out of town; but with her background as an Aboriginal Services Officer, Carol knew the ropes for contacting people and persevered in getting the help she wanted.

Not one health worker came to me and like, put me on the track to getting information or anything. The hospital didn't, nor did the health clinic that I had to go and take Malia to for weighing every week. No one. I wasn't given any pamphlets or anything. But I wanted information on what to expect, what to look for, be aware of, having a Down syndrome child. So I went asking people that had kids that were disabled. There was a couple of people that I knew in town and they told me to see the local Disability

Commission. But at that time we were in the process of transferring back to the East Kimberley so it was when I moved back here that I got in contact with the LAC and then that was it from there, she got us a fact file from the Down Syndrome Association.

In regional areas too, the assumption that assistance would be available for the asking was sometimes missing, which also limited numbers approaching the LAC.

People don't look for supports and services, they're just getting on with doing their own thing; they just don't have the need to be linked into DSC at all.[89]

The Brookton family in the East Kimberley is an example. As Wendy Brookton said, 'We were pretty independent, and we still are I suppose.' After Mark was born in 1993, the Brooktons were approached by the LAC from a regional centre in Broome (a thousand kilometres away) whenever he visited their town, maybe every couple of months. At first the family wasn't particularly interested in receiving government help, but the LAC persisted in trying to ascertain whether they had needs he could help meet, and was able to offer concrete assistance such as an airfare to facilitate attendance at a DSAWA workshop in Perth. On the whole though, the Brooktons preferred to make their own way and independently sought out speech therapy and OT as the need arose. Perth, a 3300 kilometre drive, wasn't easily accessible so they sought some help regarding early intervention from Darwin, just 820 kilometres away, and largely fell back on services and programs sent through the post, which they found 'pretty impossible' to follow. They also got information through the Down Syndrome Association in Perth.

Brenda Harvey's daughter Grace was born in Albany in 1992, and had an early visit from a DSC representative who said she was available if needed and told Brenda about the DSC library. No services or health referrals were offered though until Grace was at kindergarten, at which stage she started to access physio and speech services through DSC, but Brenda did not always find this useful. Travel was an issue, as it was for the Brooktons and other families living outside towns or where services were not offered locally. Grace also had the great advantage, from a developmental point of view, of living in an idyllic rural community with hordes of kids, lots of outdoor activities, and a wealth of community and social interaction.

> The services occasionally come here, but usually it means going to Albany [about an hour's drive away], and when she was little, it was disruptive for her. She would fall asleep on the way there and then you would have to wake her up for the appointment. I couldn't really see how beneficial it was. The speech therapy was all trips to Albany and it was a bit like a playgroup setting and singing songs and games and I just thought, well, we are doing most of this anyway, just in her everyday life because she's always had a lot of children around her to play with and a lot of talking from us.

Carol Lambert, by contrast, found community life wasn't working for her young daughter. There were no other young kids round and with school-aged children bussed off to the local town daily, life was lonely. And there were other problems.

> I know I need a lot of toys and that to build her development up. I was getting toys from the Noah's Ark Toy Library [in Perth, more than 3000 kilometres away]. They sent really

good toys, because they're very educational, but it's the hassle of keeping the toys together and sending them back. The house we are living in at the moment is cement floor, not much space for her to use them, play with and there's no other toys ...

She can play outside, but there's also cattle, they have cattle around. Our yard is a big yard with a mango tree, so they come in there, walking through that, it's so open. That's why I was hoping she would go to day care because I know they've got just the right place for her, because they've got all the toys that she might need, and it's good for her social skills. Probably be good to prepare her now for if she goes to school, so she wouldn't have any trouble there.

Even where clients are registered with their LAC, there is simply not the same access to services outside the metropolitan areas. Therapy teams visit from outside, which limits easy follow-up by parents. When Malia was three, Carol was taking her into town once every three months for hour-long sessions with therapists but while she found their intervention helpful, she felt the lack of a structured program to follow at home.

Malia's showing independence now so I think if we had a routine or a program to follow, that she could be independent herself. Since she started feeding herself she doesn't like anyone feeding her, she wants to do it herself. So I think that's a good sign, that if we do something to push her in that way, I think she'll do all right. But I don't know who to ask. I know you've got to set up a routine. So I'd be willing to do that and take up a program or something to point her in that direction. Guess we're looking out for her schooling and stuff, and probably life skills, something like that — that's for when she's older. But I think we should start now because young kids, when they're children they absorb more things.

It is also clear that in regional Western Australia people had to be much more proactive in finding information than in the metropolitan area and those like Carol Lambert who had a professional background in seeking resources were better off.

I'd say that for other people that might have a child and then don't know which way to go, there should be a lot more information placed around. I don't know, maybe at the Aboriginal Medical Services, because you just don't see much information about disabilities. I was in Derby at the time and the AMS there seemed to be a pretty good centre, but there was nothing about disabilities, nothing whatsoever.

Janet Rossi, also from regional Western Australia, acknowledged the profound impact of the absence of any support when her daughter Sandra was born in 1975. Janet's total isolation from other families in the same situation was combined with an absence of supportive services and a dearth of information — or, perhaps more correctly, a wealth of inaccurate information.

It was very difficult at first, you know, you're coming to terms with it, coming to accept it, wondering why you deserved to have a child like this and stuff like that, all these things go through your mind. I suppose I was on the verge of having a breakdown; I felt like I was the one and only, well I was at the time, that had a child like that. There was no support at all. So I just battled along with the help of my family ...

The initial diagnosis period was just so negative, like about their attitude towards Downs. I suppose they didn't know much about them to distinguish that there's mild or severe cases. They're saying that you've just got to take every day as it comes and the life span, she wasn't going to be around for long; and that they're all one level, she won't be able to learn, she won't be able to do anything and all this sort of stuff. I just sort of wondered about that because as she developed, I could see that she developed in leaps and bounds and she did learn and progress, even though she was slightly behind the normal milestones.

Living outside Perth in the 1970s and 80s, she experienced the same desolation, isolation and absence of hope women in Perth had suffered a generation previously. And like them, she set out to change things, for herself and others. At this stage, DSC was a relatively new presence in the West Kimberley and there was a real need for services.

I was one of the founding members of setting up West Kimberley Family Support [FSA]. We set that up with other families. At the time I think there was only about four of us that had children with a disability in the town. It's an incorporated group of parents of children with disabilities that come together and provide respite and support to families of children with disability, or an adult, or whatever. They engage a carer to come in and identify their needs and they get funded on their needs. I think it's now gone up to like twenty-seven people that we have, that we're providing support to.

The West Kimberley group worked alongside the LAC and other services such as Bran Nue Dae (which provides support for elderly people with disabilities), and with Home and Community Care (HACC), with these bodies all referring possible clients to the Family Support Association (FSA). Funded by DSC, the FSA provides respite for families and individuals. As Janet said, it offers the chance 'to have a break, to bring people in to give me a bit of a break, and just to meet other parents and families, share experience and support.' As her daughter grew up, Janet continued to make use of FSA for personal respite.

> Sometimes I go out to the family community at Banana Wells and stay there. I used to go up to Derby. I can still be in the house, but they are actually taking her out and they're doing things with her. Just community interaction with her, taking her shopping. She'd have her set days where she'd do different activities with them.

The Brooktons had been similarly involved in establishing a Family Support Association in the East Kimberley in the 1990s, where their focus was on funding for respite and family support, on raising community awareness of disability issues, and 'bringing communities together'. The East Kimberley region is huge, ranging from Halls Creek to Kalumburu, so bringing communities together was a mammoth task, but an essential one in terms of offering support.

Keith Brookton: We divvy the money up, where we feel the money was most needed, so it's more controlled locally. But we've taken it a little bit further than that and tried to — like with the Shire — get a disabilities plan into place and have these speakers up and try and bring the communities together.

Wendy Brookton: Yes, we all went out — a heap of people, and ladies from Warmun — and we went out camping for a weekend. It was a girls' weekend, just all girls. We went out and chatted and found some bush tucker and painted and you know just did some stuff out there. So that was really good. So it's sort of getting to know, trying to get the community a bit more — cross-culturally as well — a bit more inclusive, especially for Aboriginal people. It's pretty tough for some of the people out in the outer communities.

Carol Lambert was also involved in the East Kimberley FSA. For families in the far north, these family support associations are of more immediate benefit than the DSAWA in Perth. The DSAWA has attempted to redress this by establishing regional support contacts outside the metropolitan region, and families from these areas regularly attend Down syndrome workshops in Perth, often with the assistance of funding from DSC. But for the relatively small numbers of people with Down syndrome living in regional and remote communities and in towns far from Perth, the focus is more on community support and respite than on Down syndrome.

Whether they were in urban, rural or remote areas, every parent interviewed appreciated having services and was enormously grateful for their availability and for the people who provided them. But there is no doubt that over time, the process of being a recipient of services can sometimes become challenging. As parents became more familiar with their new child, less daunted at the idea of disability and more confident about how to manage, some aspects of having one's life turned into a timetable began to pall. Ironically too, some parents at times felt that therapists only saw their child as a disability issue.

Sometimes now I resent all that intrusion in my life and that my life wasn't as spontaneous as I thought it might be. Our days were taken up with therapy and appointments and things. They have given me great programs, they have given me good resources, good ideas but now maybe I am getting a bit territorial about his therapy. I want the time to carry them out with him myself ...

And some of the therapists, they are young, they are fresh out of uni and they don't have children of their own and I see that they are just seeing Jack as a child with Down syndrome. All their training has geared them up to look for the problems and find ways to fix the problems and sometimes I think they are finding problems where there aren't any. They expect him to sit at the table with them, people he doesn't know, do an hour of work, one activity after the other, without once throwing anything off the table or getting annoyed or getting frustrated. He is a three year old boy and I think they lose sight of that sometimes. (Britt Canning)

Parents too found themselves rewritten. At the same time as their child was being transformed into a case to be managed, parents sometimes felt they were also being redefined — from professionals, adults and parents into recipients of services. Heather Burton is a health professional herself.

I felt, I'm about to become one of my clients, what I used to see of my clients with those difficult lives, with all their problems and what have you, I was about to become one — to sort of swap sides of the fence so to speak. I've got a lot of my self-identity from being the professional, and suddenly I'm going to become the patient. So that was very, very hard.

The feeling that one's home was becoming a public space was also experienced by a number of parents. Richard Gregson captured what many parents felt, when he said that 'Sometimes it can be a bit like a revolving door at a supermarket.' For that reason, Loretta Muller was grateful for the set-up in the ACT where Cameron was born in 1989.

> They didn't come to me, we went to them and I found that better. I find it a bit invasive when people come to my house; I prefer to go out. And that was great.

All in all, it could be fairly intense. With the arrival of other children too, the dynamics of family life shift and it often becomes impossible to continue to give the child with special needs such concentrated attention. Once Mark's younger sister was born the Brooktons found it hard to keep up with the programs they had tried to set up — speech, physio and OT — and had to make decisions about what was possible within the framework of their family life. Accessing services was compounded by the fact that they lived twenty kilometres out of town on a farm and now had three young children, of whom the younger two were 'fighting, but not walking,' as the parents put it.

> I did find that it was just all too much, I mean, it was all 'Oh we're going here now; we're going there now.' It all centred around Mark and maybe his younger sister was hard done by. In the end we sort of had to make some choices about what was really important. What could we do in normal play, and what could we let slide, and what was it we really needed? Speech was probably the most important thing. In the end we went, physio? No. Most of the stuff we're doing anyway, he's bouncing on the trampoline, he gets all that sort of stuff, rather than having to go and have a little program. (Wendy Brookton)

Diana Foster was equally realistic about the need for a shift in perspective.

> I see a lot of obsessed families. I mean, it's very difficult for them to get off the topic of someone with Down syndrome and you know the stress in their family life must be enormous sometimes. Not for everyone, perhaps some can operate like that and survive it, but I certainly can't. I think there has to be a balance somewhere. The child with Down syndrome is part of the family, it can't be the whole. Perhaps we were obsessed a little bit initially. We were very keen to do all the right things and to try our hardest, but I think perhaps you get more realistic as you get more children; you can't live like that anyway, whether it's good for the child or not. I think there are some families still operating in that mode. I don't know how they keep it up for a long time, it must be very hard.

In retrospect though, as children aged, and as services declined and funds were redirected, parents recognised that the services offered had been a privilege they had not always appreciated. Helen Golding with her adopted son with Down syndrome only realised later how lucky she had been.

> Parenting children with disabilities meant that we then had therapists involved as well, which meant other people coming into the home. I knew that would happen because we had been to AIH [Authority for Intellectually Handicapped Persons] and talked about their services, but I never really appreciated the extent of that. I remember at one point saying to the people at AIH, 'Can I just have some time with this little boy on my own, without any interference?' because it seemed from day one that we had people coming in and telling me what I should and shouldn't do and what I

had to do and I needed some time just to learn to be his mum without actually having to do all of the therapy as well. But we were very lucky, in that we came in towards the end of AIH's big push on early intervention, which unfortunately they have now let go of. When I look at the level of service provision that is available now, I should have grabbed all that I could get back then. He had a social trainer right from those early months and the OT came very regularly, and the physiotherapist was there all the time.

How can the results be measured? Was our doctor right in saying that ultimately it doesn't make a difference? No one expected miracles and most parents were circumspect about the outcomes of therapy. Pamela Franklin, for instance, was modest about her daughter's achievements and her own role in helping her attain them, saying, 'I don't know if it paid off. She is very good communication wise and things like that, so whether or not that helped, I suppose we will never know.' Similarly Diana Foster said, 'John speaks very well. He reads. He's got a lot of skills that I'm very happy with, you know, for his age. Whether he would have done that or not, I don't know.' But Luke Middleton had no doubts whatsoever about the value of services.

Within a month of Laura's birth she had the services of a psychologist, a speech therapist, an occupational therapist, a physiotherapist and two social trainers. I thought they were fantastic. It wasn't just that they did great work with Laura but they taught us what to do as well. I came to believe that the more work you do with a child the better the results will be and I am convinced that Laura did so well because of their work.

Helen Golding's experience with adoption puts her in a better position than most to assess whether or not it makes a difference. When the family adopted Josie in 1989 when she was aged two and a half, she had been living in a foster home since birth and had not received any therapy services. The results were palpable: 'She was a long way delayed at two and half compared to where Damian and Charlotte were at two and half.' According to Helen, at that stage when Family and Community Services (FCS) fostered out children with Down syndrome the children were referred to AIH for services, but FCS did not insist on their accessing it.

> I had the argument with AIH several times, before Josie even came to us, that as far as I was concerned this child's therapy needs were being neglected. Their attitude was that while she was in the care of those people, we had to do what they wanted, and if they didn't want us to be there providing a service then we couldn't be there. I tried to convince the foster mother that she needed to put some pressure on AIH to get a social trainer to come in and work with Josie because she really wasn't making progress, but I don't think she could cope with doing any more than she was doing. While the day-to-day care was fine and the kids certainly had lots of love and affection, Josie needed more than that and she wasn't getting it.

Whether or not one's child has a disability, parents generally aspire to do everything they reasonably can to enhance their child's development and future prospects. Therapies and services added a compounding element to that equation. As Loretta Muller said, 'The therapy sessions certainly did me a power of good' at a time when the future looked bleak, and few if any families would disagree with Trish Weston's comment: 'It was a lot of hard work. But it was right for us at the time, I think, to do that.'

On a global basis, the availability of early intervention and general services in the lives of people with Down syndrome and their families has led to outcomes in terms of realising individual potential undreamed of by parents in the early postwar years. International shifts in attitudes to intellectual disability and the emergence of doctrines which highlighted the potency of training and skill development, the commitment of parent-based support organisations such as the DSAWA and the role of the state in providing services cannot be overestimated. Together they continue to raise expectations and generate hope.

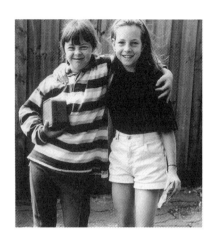

chapter 5

LEARNING TO BE NORMAL, LEARNING TO BE DISABLED

'It wasn't a great year for us basically. It was probably as hard for us to take as it was when we actually found out that Will had Down syndrome.'
(Trish Weston on her child's first year in the school system)

'I said to him, "Well, you do know that I can actually bring him down on the first day of grade one and say, here you are?" and he said, "Yes, and I can sit him in the corner for six months and he will do nothing, then you will have to move him."'
(Helen Golding)

'He's learnt how to be normal, if you know what I mean, and I think that's the biggest thing that being in an included environment like that gives you.'
(Alison Austen)

'I graduated in year twelve and that was it, I was in the future.'
(Rebecca Innes)

The baby comes home, and life goes on. But then it is time to think about school. For some parents, sending a child with a disability off to school at the age of five or so becomes the catalyst for a philosophical assessment of the whole meaning of disability, prompting the need to evaluate what sort of a life they want for their child, in terms which the parents of other children, facing no more taxing decision than whether to go private or public, might find hard to understand. Education is one of the most fraught areas for parents of a child with a disability and there are few topics which generate more heat or cause more pain. The school years, bridging the gap between childhood and adult life, are about more than just the process of formal education. As the child with a disability negotiates the transition from the safe haven of the home into the larger community, parents are forced to confront, once again, the significance of disability in terms of friendship, social and recreational opportunities and acceptance.

Since my daughter Maddie was born in 1992, Western Australians have seen a huge number of changes in schooling options for kids with intellectual disabilities, ranging from special schools to educational support centres and units, to supported full inclusion, though the opportunity to access some of those is still dependent on where one lives. While integration in a mainstream state school classroom had been a theoretical possibility for children since 1984, in practice this option was available to very few people with intellectual disabilities until the start of the twenty-first century when a report issued by the state government promised a number of new 'pathways' to a future of more inclusive schooling.

Inclusion is the holy grail to which many parents of a child with Down syndrome aspire, at least at some stage in their child's life. Some pursue it relentlessly, sometimes at significant emotional cost; others decide that it is a poisoned chalice and follow a different path. This chapter explores some of the educational opportunities available to Western Australian children over the past few decades and examines the conflicts and resolutions which emerge when the choices offered by the educational system clash with parents' views about what is best for their child. As one parent of a child with severe disabilities put it in a submission to the 2004 state government report on education for children with disabilities, 'coping with a child with ... disabilities can be exhausting and no parent welcomes the added grief of having to battle the system to achieve what is best for their child.'[90] Yet parents of older people with Down syndrome would undoubtedly have welcomed the opportunity to battle, and the chance to agonise over choices. For them, there were none.

After a year or so attending a class run through what became the Spastic Welfare Association, Trevor Simpson started in a special class at the local primary school. It was the early 1950s; Trevor was about eight years old and was in a small pioneering cohort of children with Down syndrome whose parents had not institutionalised them. But having made that decision, his parents faced the consequences of limited support and educational facilities. His mother Mavis recalled that there were just over a dozen students in the class, run by one woman.

They were, you know, completely different types of children. Different levels of ability and it was a very much of a hotchpotch and they were only tolerated by the school really; they weren't given any particular help. And she was just a person with a lot of tolerance and understanding, but no special skills, and there was no thought of teaching Trevor to read, he didn't really speak to any degree there at that time.

Trevor stayed there for about three or four years and then moved on to Minbalup Education Centre for Slow Learning Children in Harper Street, Victoria Park, which opened in 1954.

It was mostly activities to improve their manual dexterity and that type of thing. They didn't do any real reading, or number work, but it was, I suppose, a modified form of a special class program and they had a lot of outdoor activities. He thoroughly enjoyed that, and of course going in the bus. The group got two little Austin vans and I used to drive one of those when it first started. Oh, for quite a while, I did, and we would pick up a busload of children and take them there, and he enjoyed that.

At Minbalup, Mavis was given to understand that Trevor wouldn't be able to learn to read or write 'or anything of that sort'. From that beginning, and in the face of those expectations, Trevor went on to gain quite extensive written skills and a fascination for language — but he was very much a self-taught man.

At first it was all sight reading. He was interested in the television, of course, and the television programs, but he gradually acquired some phonics and he can read fairly well, but he'll stumble on unexpected words and he doesn't always grasp the meaning of what he is reading. He's got a fascination with dictionaries and encyclopaedias. He gets interested in a word or some idea and he'll look it up. He's also very religious. He's always typing out what I suppose you'd call statements of his beliefs or something and they're always in very stilted language, because he looks up a word in the dictionary and finds the meaning for it and uses that lovely big word.

Trevor was in the vanguard of children with Down syndrome who were kept at home with their parents rather than institutionalised and actually provided with some education, albeit focused more on training than literacy. Previously no education or support services had been offered at all. By the 1960s however, as deinstitutionalisation began in earnest and as children increasingly remained with their families, a more systematic approach to the education of children with disabilities emerged. By the mid 1970s, in addition to SLCG day activity centres, there were sixty special education classes in primary schools, twenty-three in secondary schools and fourteen training centres.[91] Some of the students in those special classes would have had Down syndrome.

Within a few years of Trevor's school experience, some teachers were becoming more prepared — often in the face of ridicule from their peers — to recognise that kids with Down syndrome and other disabilities were capable of learning and deserved the right to be taught in the classroom. Geoffrey Mann was lucky enough to find such a teacher. After a disastrous start at a special school in Fremantle, Irrabeena helped his parents find a place for Geoffrey in a small preschool for kids with disabilities, and a subsequent placement at Millen School.

Millen had its ups and downs but fortunately for Geoffrey, it had one teacher who was dedicated to the idea that these people could be taught something other than wiping down the tables and sweeping the floor. In fact, she was bet in the staffroom that she couldn't teach that stupid Geoffrey Mann to read. She said, I'll take you on. And it took her two weeks to get Geoffrey started on reading. And I was so impressed with her endeavours that I got involved in working in the classroom as an unpaid aide, as a volunteer aide, and I used to bring about eight or ten ladies over to the school every Monday morning so that in that classroom every child virtually had one-to-one attention for a couple of hours to start the week off with a good push. It was really amazing the success that particular teacher had with literacy and numeracy training which, at that stage, was still controversial within the special schools. A lot of teachers wouldn't have a bar of it — you couldn't be expected to teach these people that sort of skill. (Muriel Mann)

Muriel's story, like Mavis's, underlines how dependent the special schools were on parents — typically mothers — for extra help, such as assistance in classrooms and driving buses. Geoffrey was also fortunate in that his family had an academic background; their expectations for him were framed by the belief that he should have the opportunity to learn, and they were prepared to advocate on behalf of him and other kids with disabilities.

I didn't see that he should be specifically excluded from being taught just because he was Down syndrome. That was the attitude of many teachers at the time. In fact, they were still excluding children from special schools if they weren't toilet-trained or they couldn't climb the steps — flimsy pretexts for exclusion! (Muriel Mann)

Mavis Simpson, Muriel Mann and other women like them became involved in the Slow Learning Children's Group which played an important role in initiating change in the 1960s and 70s.

Children like Geoffrey were educated in segregated 'special school' settings, but by the 1980s, new ideas about integrating or mainstreaming children with disabilities within ordinary classrooms and schools were emerging. The Beazley report into education in Western Australia (1984) advocated that 'handicapped ... children ... should be integrated as far as is possible into the normal or usual school setting,' which meant special 'units' for children with intellectual disabilities incorporated within the normal school setting and the integration of children into the regular classroom where possible, alongside the continuation of special education centres for those with more severe disabilities.[92] It also recognised the need for additional training and resourcing for classroom teachers and, in line with the 1978 British government Warnock report into the education of handicapped children, advocated that children should be grouped on the basis of their educational needs rather than according to their medical condition or disability label.[93]

The Beazley report was followed in 1993 by the Shean report into the education of children with disabilities, which went a step further to advocate the beginning of a process of integration.[94] This was initially little more than what would now be described as 'main-dumping', namely placing children in some mainstream classes without adequate resources to facilitate their social inclusion, but in the following decade in Western Australia, a scheme was introduced to enable a handful of primary school children with intellectual disabilities such as Down syndrome — fewer than a dozen each year — to apply for a fully funded inclusive place in a regular state school, with the funding and inclusion package to remain with the child throughout their school life. Early in the twenty-first century, following that trial, inclusion in government schools was to be made available to all students with an intellectual disability who wanted it, while the older facilities of education support schools, units and centres were to remain for those who felt their child needed them.

While policy shifts underlined the emergence of new possibilities, the reality of choice didn't always trickle down into the classroom. People entering the educational system in the late 1980s and the 1990s, when these changes should have been developing real teeth, sometimes found themselves still powerless in negotiations within the educational system; at other times though, they found surprisingly positive opportunities in a particular school, even if it hadn't always been their first choice for their child.

The principal's attitude was often the key. Cameron Danes' family in Albany in the 1990s had an excellent experience with his primary schooling, even though it was not as inclusive as his parents might have wished.

> We were very lucky, we had two really good principals. The ed. support principal when we first arrived, and the primary school principal was very innovative and was wanting to make this the best school in the universe, and it was really great, and part of that was to include the kids with disabilities. I think our school is quite novel in its approach to what we do. I know when our principal used to go to meet with other principals they would be amazed at what we did. That was really good. (Loretta Muller)

More typical however was dissatisfaction. In 1988 Helen Golding started looking at educational options for her son Damian. She thought the local state primary school with its education support unit would be ideal, and phoned the principal.

His response was, 'No, we don't have kids like that at this school,' and I said, 'Well, what sort of children *do* you have in your unit?' 'Oh we don't have kids with *those* sorts of problems.' Being a little informed as to what the system was, I said to him, 'Well you do know that I can actually bring him down on the first day of grade one and say, here you are,' and he said, 'Yes, and I can sit him in the corner for six months and he will do nothing, then you will have to move him' ...

The school psychologist contacted me and said, 'That is atrocious! He shouldn't have said that!' But as it happened, the way the system was working at that point, the principal *was* allowed to do that. He could say, 'I will not have these children in my school.' ...

The education support unit was a class of children with learning difficulties, but he didn't want children with disabilities. Eventually his hand was forced and he had to take them, but he still wouldn't take mine. The psychologist said to me, 'Look, if you really want to we can force the issue and we can make him take your son,' and I said, 'I don't want to put my son into a school where he is not wanted and if that is the principal's attitude, then a teacher who is prepared to go the extra distance is going to have no support so there is no point; I would rather find somewhere where he is going to be wanted.'

In the early 1990s Diana Foster also encountered difficulties. Her son John had completed pre-primary at one local primary school, but she wanted him to continue at a different local school.

At the end of the school year, we tried to get him into another school, which has a satellite classroom in it, but it turned into a nightmare. The principal was initially quite supportive of the idea. We'd started consultation earlier in the year, and seen him on about three or four occasions, and it was all set up for John to start school that next year. Then in December he called us and said, 'I've changed my mind. He can't come.' And so we went, 'Oh, what! You've changed your mind?' And he said, 'Oh, he needs a full-time aide. He hasn't got an aide, so he can't come.' Which was wonderful! It was typical of what he turned out to be like! He's since been removed from the school for the same sorts of tactics.

Looking for a school for their daughter in 1995, Laura Middleton's parents' first choice was the local primary school where her sister was already enrolled, and which she had visited in her stroller almost daily from the week she was born. The family was ideologically committed to state schooling and to inclusion and had tried to get Laura into the small-scale new educational inclusion plan then being trialled in the state, which included full aide support.

They were offering something like seven included places across the state that year and we didn't get one. So we spoke to the principal at the local primary school. 'Well if we could get an aide,' he said, 'but quite frankly if we don't get an aide, as a matter of justice to the other kids I can't have her here.' So that was that. (Jude Lawrence)

How hard was it to get an aide? When talking to a principal it was essential to present the child in as positive a light as possible to encourage the school to look favourably on the prospect of their attending; yet when it came time to write the aide application — if it got that far — the child had to be presented in the least favourable light possible, with any strengths played down, a classic Catch 22. This was a game most families initially despised but eventually accepted as the reality of the system, and learned the rules. Many would continue playing for a very long time.

Loretta Muller discovered this when inquiring about applying for an aide for her son Cameron.

> They actually said to me Cameron wouldn't get one because he wasn't a flight risk, he was toilet-trained, he was too good for an aide! ... But despite his capabilities, they were really not very encouraging, they didn't really want us to come there. I felt they were really under-staffed and that they probably weren't doing as good a job as they would like and they recommended that I go to the centre.

Within the state educational system, possibilities for Laura Middleton — like Cameron, toilet-trained, not a wanderer, and with the principal of her local school not prepared to admit her without an aide — were also limited.

> There was a special ed. unit at another school up the road and we were told to go there. Well, we had a look. Laura at the age of five would have been in the same classroom with huge big boys of twelve and thirteen, who had absolutely nothing in common with her except that they had a disability, a different sort of disability. She wasn't allowed to be part of the mainstream classroom until she got to grade three or four because, they said, it was 'too confusing' for the children to be joined in with the regular classes. It was physically isolated from the rest of the school. It was just horrible, and yet it's supposed to be good. (Jude Lawrence)

So the family went independent.

In 2000 another family reacted almost identically to a very similar encounter with the state system. Shannon da Silva had been in an inclusive setting at school in the United Kingdom since she was three and her parents had thoroughly researched the educational options available in Western Australia before they arrived. They were adamant that special education was not for them.

We were aware that there *was* inclusion, which was what we wanted. But it was quite hard to get and most places had this education support unit and it sounded like special education to us! When we arrived and were pushed in the direction of one of these special ed. units straightaway, we went along to see it, though we really didn't think we were going to be interested; and sure enough, we got there and we were pretty much horrified, actually. I mean, they talked all the time about integration, but the special education unit was in a different building from the rest of the school, tucked away around the corner, and the children with special needs were in this unit every morning and were only allowed into some sort of regular classroom in the afternoon when they were doing craft and things like that that they could cope with. And they had like the whole gamut, right across the age range from the whole school, in this one room. And it was — I mean, it was a tiny room, with no windows or anything, so it wasn't a very *pleasing* environment. I just remember envisaging Shannon in this room and thinking, 'Absolutely no way! Over my dead body!'

So we bypassed that completely and went to the local primary school in the area we thought we might be living. And we said, 'We don't want the school with the special ed. unit. We want Shannon to be in a regular primary school. That's where she has been until now.' And the principal said, 'Well, we wouldn't have any funding for it and we can't really cope with it.' And although I know it is our right to put our child wherever we want, we both felt that the biggest factor in successful inclusion is the child being wanted. So there was absolutely no point in trying to turn somebody around at the point where they are already clearly saying, 'We don't want this child.' I am never going to do that. I would home-school my child rather than put them in a school where they are not wanted. It has to be a school that is going to say, 'Yes, we accept this child, we want this child, and we are sure that she can learn here.' (Karen Langley)

In the following pages, the experiences of five individuals who each faced different sorts of choices — James Austen, Georgia Robb, Jack Canning, Lucy Burton and Rebecca Innes — are related in some depth to illustrate the complexities of the educational process and how very different the experience was for individual families. Their circumstances also underline that even after an initial decision was made about schooling, the process was seldom straightforward.

The Austens were relatively satisfied with the direction they chose, which fitted in well with their parenting philosophy of giving their youngest son James, born in 1989, experiences as close as possible to those his two brothers had enjoyed. While they appreciated that it was not entirely perfect, they kept to their chosen path and for most of the time James's mother Alison was pleased with the outcome.

We just wanted to live a normal family life. James swam like his brothers, he played footy like his brothers did, he went to the same school and wore their uniforms — handed down, one, two, three! We just wanted James to live a life of joy and involvement in everything around him.

The first choice we made was for James to go to Montessori where he would get a good grounding in those early years. The Montessori set-up is just so good in the sense that it enhances the way people with Down syndrome learn really. Then in year one, we went to our local Catholic primary school. We decided that we'd like James to go to the same school as his brothers, so that we could be in touch with local families ...

Looking back, there came a point where perhaps we could have looked for something different. We did think about it, but James was very highly regarded by staff and by the other students and the other families, so we felt as though we belonged. But as James got older, he was surrounded by people who accepted him but there was not really any one-to-one friendship, so we sought that in other places.

Education-wise the onus is always on the family to ensure that things were happening, and while they were responsive, you sort of had to keep your finger on the pulse all the time. We always followed it up and pursued a bit more. But as time went on I think we came to the realisation that it was more important that James enjoyed where he was and that he was positive about things than for us to be pushing him down a track that he really didn't want. So we just let him be and he blossomed a bit more ...

I think he was happy at school. He had good times and he had hard times too. He always gets back to how stubborn he was. I said, 'But why were you stubborn?' He said, 'It was hard' ... He made it hard for teachers, in the sense he had everything there and people wanting to help him and he refused it a lot of the time. They used to have to coax things out of him. I think he knew what he was doing. He was resisting, wanting to find his own path even then. We were trying to push him in a direction I suppose, but only from the point of view that we wanted him to get the most out of schooling and prepare himself for a more independent life. That's always what's been behind it.

He had an aide, yes, for a few hours, of a morning mainly. Other than that he was just one of the guys. I think that's been positive; but there have been negatives as well in the sense that there were times when he'd be sitting on his own, and there were times when someone might say something not nice to him. But yes, I think the positives far outweighed the negative.

The whole set-up of being in a school in our local community and families knowing him and being part of the community, all of that has had a very positive spin-off with James because I think he's learnt how to be normal, if you know what I mean, and I think that's the biggest thing that being in an included environment like that gives you.

After primary school the family opted for James to continue to follow the same route as his brothers and to attend a local co-ed Catholic secondary college, where he was enrolled in an education support unit but attending some mainstream classes. It was this combination which attracted Georgia Robb's parents to the same school a few years later. For Alison, James's high school experience was mostly positive, though going from a regular classroom to a unit was a thought-provoking experience for them both.

The last couple of years maybe of primary school, I think, were harder, they were probably the hardest for James. So when you get to the College, it was very exciting and it was also a bit of a relief. I think I felt, aha, I don't have to keep going from year to year giving the message about what James needs. He was going to be in a place [the education support unit] where someone would follow through with him. But also the College I think has a good feel about the place too. Our other boys really loved it. The students seemed to be very relaxed and there's a good sort of rapport between students and teachers. I think for James that was a very positive environment. He loved being out there with the guys and he seemed to gravitate to the really popular boys in his mainstream class. He'd come home saying, 'Oh so-and-so's really cool.' So that was a really nice thing ...

He'd never been part of a unit before though, and so then we had to take on board being with a whole lot of other people who have a disability as well. That was quite a learning experience for James. I remember in the very early years he came home and I questioned him about his day, and had he made some new friends, and what are they like and all this. He'd say, 'Oh a bit strange.' 'What do you mean, a bit strange?' 'Mmm, skinny legs!' Some funny things came out but he was really trying to deal with people looking and behaving perhaps a bit differently to what he'd been used to. So that was quite a different experience for him. He had to learn how to be disabled, I suppose ...

I think he could see that he was able to get more help with his school work, but we were more interested in that than he was. The best parts of school for him were the outings and doing things with his friends.

James was also an excellent swimmer, representing the school in open events, and trained with the team throughout his school years, which undoubtedly enhanced his social inclusion. Andrew Danes similarly recognised the value of sport for his son Cameron in Albany.

> He's got a nice group of friends, some nice boys in his class that will look out for him. He is very much into sports. He has always done well and they have included him in all kind of sports on weekends as well.

Gender — growing up as 'one of the boys' — may also have been a factor in James's successful high school experience. Pamela Franklin found socialisation and peer support less successful for her teenage daughter at an all-girls Catholic high school and it does seem that being 'one of the girls' can be harder.

> Socialisation has been the main problem. She *is* different and I can't deny that. She can't keep up now and it became more and more apparent as she got older. For instance, now her peers are talking about boys and they go off and do things by themselves and she can't do that. She can't talk on the same level as them. So, I am pragmatic enough to know that that is going to be a problem and that she is probably going to need people at her own level as friends — but I don't know why a so-called normal person couldn't have somebody like Catherine as a friend. They wouldn't be a friend in the sense of their other friends, but they could still be a friend if you like. I suppose that would be my ultimate dream that she would have people who would like her for who she is, even though she was different, but that doesn't even happen with kids who are 'normal' who are a little bit different.

Despite James's successful social experience at the College, by the time he reached year eleven the Austen family's satisfaction with the College was evaporating fast. By that stage he was already doing two days a week work experience and TAFE, in school time, but a personality clash with one of the teachers in the education support unit 'made his life a misery.' James's experience shows how even the best situations can sometimes change. In the end the family decided to persevere.

I think the last two years were very difficult for him. There weren't many other options and a change at that late stage seemed like too big an upheaval for him personally. There was no easy answer. He loved the school, his friends, mainstream connections, being part of the school swimming team, but it left us with a bad taste in our mouths and not a totally happy ending for James. In the end he was glad to leave and we were glad it was all over. We were just marking time so he could complete his last year, graduate with his classmates, be presented with the school colours which was a real honour for him. We couldn't deny him all that! It only goes to show how teachers can 'make or break' the situation sometimes. (Alison Austen)

Like James, Georgia Robb (born 1993) started school at the age of three when she was enrolled at an early intervention program for children with disabilities. After completing kindy, she attended the local Catholic primary school where she and another little girl of the same age were fully supported in mainstream classes. Her mother Virginia already had a special relationship with the school — she taught there.

I was pretty pushy as far as getting her accepted, and also she got a lot of support. She had an excellent teacher assistant, who was with her nearly the whole seven years and she's just brilliant and Georgia was mainstream the whole way.

By the time she had completed primary school Georgia had reasonable social skills and acceptable literacy and numeracy, though 'her speech is very poor; she understands a lot more than people think because she gets what's going on, but she can't always communicate.'

Like the Austens, her parents chose to send her to the local Catholic college with many of her primary school friends; it was also where her elder siblings had gone. Georgia was enrolled in the education support unit there, and Virginia believed it would be a fruitful environment for her because it seemed to offer a continuation of the mainstream opportunities she had enjoyed at primary school as well as educational support in core areas. Soon though, the Robbs began to experience difficulties with the school because of the quality of the education offered within the support unit.

The kids in the ed. support unit do their own literacy and numeracy, but then they go over to the mainstream school for their electives and those sort of things; that's generally I understood how it worked, and they had their mainstream home room. So they're mixing with the mainstream kids every day. Home room, religion and electives; and then their four core subjects they do in the ed. support unit. I thought that was the ideal way to go.

And she was in a very, very good cohort at her primary school, they were a really good bunch of kids and most of them were going to the College, so my initial feeling was that it was really important for her to go through with kids that she had good relationships with ...

And initially we were happy, she was happy there. Her friends that she was in primary school with, quite a few of them were in her home room. But towards the end of year eight, I started to have a few concerns because I wasn't seeing any accountability of programming. I was concerned about the lack of assessment; I suppose being a teacher myself and also the fact that I have taught children with special needs, I was concerned in terms of literacy and numeracy. It just seemed very ad hoc to me and the programs I was given, they were rubbish basically. By year nine, nothing was changing, I felt that I wasn't being heard and I had had a couple of interviews with the head of the ed. support unit.

It got to the stage also where Georgia was not happy. I think basically that she was frustrated; she knows what it means to work hard and she wasn't doing any work. I feel that a lot of the work, there's no content to it, it was just fill-in kind of work. I couldn't see any progress in her literacy and numeracy. Her literacy had gone backwards.

The fact that Georgia was getting more and more unhappy was really probably what made us decide to pull her out. She was just crying every night. She was coming home and she wasn't happy. It was very hard to find out what was going on at school. She's not hugely verbal, but we know her well enough to know she wasn't happy.

The family decided to make a change to a local high school with an education support centre which, unlike an education support unit, is 'a totally separate funded school, but it's on the main grounds of the main school. So they have their own principal, their own administration.'

The thing that probably persuaded me was the very first time I went in to see the principal, he said, 'Would you like to see our programs?' and he had printed out their whole ed. support unit programs with the literacy, the numeracy, the home room, how everything worked and it was transparent, fluent and accountable, and that was a really good thing for me.

We just haven't looked back, it's brilliant. The school she's at now, she wants to go to school every single day, including in the holidays and on the weekends, so that tells me that she's having a pretty good time.

Virginia was well aware that philosophically she had done a complete about face in terms of what sort of educational system she wanted for her daughter. She and her husband Alan had initially chosen the College because it appeared to offer the educational benefits of a separate setting for core subjects, in addition to the social benefits of the mainstream environment. But as far as they were concerned, the mainstreaming in electives appeared to be little more than 'main-dumping'. It certainly was nothing like the inclusion she had hoped for.

Like for example, she did jewellery and, of course, the teacher is trying to get twenty other kids through the jewellery program to assess them and have something for them to learn by the end of the semester; well Georgia is not going to be high on his priority list because he's got all these other kids. So she sits in the corner and does something that's a bit tokenistic, and there's no learning.

While the education support students at Georgia's new school are not integrated with other mainstream students, as far as Virginia is concerned the educational and social benefits are substantial.

They have mainstream teachers, they access the tuckshop, they have their little area that they hang out in near the tuckshop, just like the year twelves and the year elevens and everybody else. The principal said something really interesting to me: 'All teenage kids are tribal, and they will go to their groups, to their little tribes, whatever type of group there is, and the ed. support kids are no different.' They're happy to hang out with the kids in their group, because they can communicate with them, they've got a relationship. There's no problems with the mainstream kids, they're not picked on or isolated or anything like that, they're just accepted as part of the school community.

And she's got friends. There's a couple of friends that have Saturday afternoon soirees and they go and all hang out together.

Georgia now has a large circle of school friends with whom, like many teenagers, she spends a good portion of her weekends. While there have been no mainstream friendships generated through the new high school, Virginia recognised that this was probably not going to happen in the educationally segregated environment; but they had not developed anyway at the College, despite the ostensible 'mainstreaming'. And did she miss that opportunity for Georgia?

No, I don't. We are in a great community here, so where we live we've got lots of friends around the neighbourhood that Georgia hangs out with. I'm not sorry about giving up [on inclusion] any more. It was a hard decision and it's not something I initially thought I would be happy with. But looking at it now, in hindsight, I think it's a far better way to go.

Britt Canning came to a similar conclusion though for slightly different reasons. When I first interviewed Britt in

1999, four year old Jack had started at the local kindy and both he and his mother were delighted with it. Early intervention, and the work Britt had done in taking Jack to activities and play sessions with other children paid clear dividends in Jack's excellent classroom behaviour. Britt was especially taken with the teacher's attitude.

> I rang to see about getting him a place. And she said, 'Oh, I have never had the privilege of teaching a child with Down syndrome but I just can't wait to meet him, bring him in.' He has got an aide, although they reckon that the aide really should be there for some of the other kids. And actually the teacher pulled me aside last term and said, 'There are actually a couple of kids in this group we consider to be a little bit more *special* than Jack,' which is quite funny.

> He loved it from day one. He had been used to workshops and that sort of structure of sitting down and working, and sitting down to listen to a story or doing music, and they were surprised. I think they expected him to maybe try and do a runner or be disruptive during story time, but he is perfect; he sits there and takes it all in.

Even when Jack was as young as four, though, Britt recognised that developmental differences were already leading to social differences in the playground.

> I went up there one day and I was dropping him off and just thought I would hang around as I left, outside the gate. And it did break my heart a bit. He was on his own and he was in the boat and he was just very much in his own world and the other kids were all mixing and it did bring home to me the gap that ever widens and I felt sad for him.

Helen Golding had observed the same thing at her son's preschool some years earlier.

I really didn't have anyone in the family I could directly compare him with and I was basically looking at this child on his own and he seemed to be doing really well in isolation. Then I went and did the mother's roster at pre-primary and was absolutely horrified at the gap, the size of the gap between him and the other kids. The other kids were wonderful with him, they were very good, they were very patient but the distance between where his abilities were and where their abilities were was just huge.

Though Britt had her reservations, she remained committed to the idea of inclusion. The next step for Jack was to be a small independent Anglican school.

They do accept children with special needs but they don't have a special ed. unit. So they are mainstream, which sounds great in theory but it is only good if you get the support he needs and he keeps learning and he has got friends. I do worry about that. I would like to get some advice from other people though. See how integration really does work. *If* it does work.

Some years later I caught up with Jack and Britt again. Jack had completed kindy and pre-primary at government schools, then moved on as planned to the local Anglican school; but, as Britt explained, he subsequently left that school to attend an education support centre attached to a state primary school.

When he was in year four [at the Anglican school], his teacher, who I respect very much, was honest, and she said to me, 'He's just not coping.' I suspect now that he was becoming depressed. I was getting calls at lunchtime to pick him up; he'd fallen asleep at his desk. The kids were great, they were really lovely kids. The staff did everything they could, and he had a full-time aide by that stage, a full-time experienced teacher assistant, although that took a few years to get that happening. He was on his own program. But I think that what he lacked in the end was a peer group and they couldn't provide that for him.

Inclusion was one of the things Britt had sought for Jack at that school but as the years had gone by, her views had shifted.

It was a matter of me letting go of something that I wanted, but in the end that wasn't important, it was about Jack. I wanted to do what was best for Jack and I'd read all these reports and spoken to lots of people and yes, the big thing out there is inclusion, and inclusion in the mainstream. But I've changed my definition of inclusion now, because really Jack wasn't included there, because he was sitting away from the other children; he was becoming disruptive, so they had to move him away physically. He couldn't relate to what was going on in the classroom, it meant nothing to him. Even though he had his own work to do, he wasn't part of a group. Year one was his only good year, when I look back. Yes, I should have moved him out. But then the school sort of came forward at that point, because things were getting tough in year two and, 'No worries, we've got a special ed. teacher coming in to teach year three.' They were very supportive, but in a way it made it harder for me to leave.

In the end however, Jack's clear unhappiness left Britt with no option and she began to consider the alternatives to inclusive schooling.

I'd heard good things about the ed. support centre at the state primary school. Went out to have a look, took Jack with us, my husband Peter came as well, and yes, he was in there two weeks later. Jack just took to it, that was the big thing. He didn't want to leave that day we went to visit. Almost overnight, happier, healthier, learning more, talking more. They do manage to engage him all day long. I've seen his timetable, and they work really hard, but he's thoroughly enjoying it, because it's all designed for him. The principal is fantastic, she's very proactive, a very strong leader, and the staff — they're brilliant out there. It's got a great atmosphere, the kids are happy, and he's very happy. Where he is now, he's part of a class, the children are working at a similar level to him. He participates from the minute he gets in there to the minute he leaves; he's doing something all day long.

Socially as well, Britt noticed changes in her son.

At the other school I think he was playing more and more on his own as time went by, even though the other children were nice to him — and certainly there was no teasing or bullying going on — he was almost the class pet, I think; everyone wanted to look after him and do stuff for him. There was a certain amount of kudos attached to that among the kids, which is positive, but in the end it wasn't very good for Jack, because he wasn't becoming independent. He wasn't socialising on an equal footing. Whereas when he went to the ed. support centre, there was still a certain element of mothering going on among a couple of the girls — Jack just seems to attract that. But he can communicate better with the kids. I've seen him actually have conversations with some of these children.

Yes, I do have a few regrets with Jack. I know I did what I thought was best at the time, so I try not to hammer myself too much, but if I had my time again ...

But it's never too late because we've noticed a big difference. Even though his speech is poor he's definitely a lot more social now, a lot more confident. Just the way he walks into that school, so much more independent. I drop him off out the front now, I don't even get out of the car, I'm not allowed to. He walks himself in. His shoulders are back, he's just so proud of himself. Packs his own school bag, makes his own bed. They demand that, they have very high expectations, realistically high expectations of what he can do. Whereas where he was, he had a class full of mothers, everybody doing for him, and assuming that he couldn't do things for himself, when he was very capable.

Britt reflected on her own growth too, as well as her son's.

I guess I've learnt to be quite flexible now, and not be afraid to make changes. Because I think I became so dogmatic, and it had almost become a bit of a crusade. I was going to all these inclusions workshops. I was at that school every second week for a meeting, or problem solving. We'd come up with all these great ideas and were putting them into practice. To start with I met with a bit of resistance, but I think I convinced them. I guess I was working hard at it and they saw that. So they came to the party as well, and they provided the aide.

They did everything they could; without actually providing him with a class of six children working at his level, there was nothing more they could do. It was just time. I knew that time would come, but I had hoped he would see out primary school. But he was definitely getting to the point ... when he was there, he was falling asleep; he didn't want to be there.

However, Britt was careful not to universalise her experience with Jack.

Don't get me wrong, I'm not anti-inclusion in the mainstream, I'm just pro-choice, and for all those choices to be presented as equally valid. I felt that if I moved him out of mainstream I would be failing in some way. But in the end it's up to individual families, what schools are around, what suits that individual child, what your own expectations are. I've got friends whose kids are in mainstream classes and they're doing fine.

Lucy Burton is just such a kid. Her mother Heather was adamant that for her, inclusive education was the only possible option. What she expected for her daughter at primary school was exposure to the full range of the curriculum, and she got it. When I asked Heather whether she would have considered a different educational environment for Lucy, she was very clear about the reasons for her choice.

I am fully aware that a lot of that was about my baggage and my feeling of stigmatisation about special schools, and also my desperation for my daughter to be part of a community, to not be ostracised, stereotyped, segregated. A lot of people have said I've gone the hard road of inclusion, where you have to constantly work and problem solve, whatever, but to go into a segregated setting would have been a lot harder for me. I couldn't have faced it; and I would have been battling with them every step of the way because I don't think they would have offered the education that I expect her to have.

I've got some great examples: Lucy coming to me in year four and talking about the pyramids and how they were built, and the Egyptians and all that. I just felt that if she was in year four in a special school she would have been going, 'Look Mum, I've pasted this onto this.' But then you ask yourself, well, what use is that to her, when it may well be that come the end of year twelve, she will not need to know about the Egyptians or anything else. But that's actually the case for every student ...

She's just done a project on chlorine; she did a project on drought. She's done a project on ancient civilisations and she came to me and said, 'Mum, I've decided I'm not going to do the Egyptians, we did that in year four; I'm going to do the Aztecs.' Now I think that's fantastic. It gives her conversation topics and while her conversation is not like other people's, I still think that her language skills and social skills are pretty darn good compared to what they might be if she hadn't had that kind of stimulation. And I've often had teachers say, 'Lucy is better at some things than some of the other kids.' And it was a real lesson for them!

With Lucy's inclusive primary schooling being such a positive experience, her parents chose her high school very carefully. One option was a co-educational Catholic secondary college for which Lucy's primary was a feeder school, so that was a fairly obvious choice. But for Heather, the fact that it had an education support centre was a negative feature. While some parents who opted for education support saw the emphasis on life skills as a plus, for Heather it was totally at odds with what she wanted for her daughter. Another possibility was a state secondary school but for a number of reasons, Lucy's parents were initially not keen.

It was a massive school and everything, and I thought it was a bit daunting. But as soon as we went there, we felt different. They were like, 'Look we're here to give Lucy the best education we can; we'll offer this support, that support. This is what we're about.' It was just a whole different ball game. I talked to people who had kids with disabilities and I talked to the aides. And you see, they hadn't really had a kid like mine at the school before, with an intellectual disability. But they've been fantastic ...

So she's totally mainstream. In some ways her needs are not always met ... they have a science lesson and it goes straight over her head, but some of the teachers know just how to wangle things. So for instance in French — I think Lucy's learnt more French in six months than she learnt in all her years of Italian at primary school, because the teacher just gets it. She just asks the question in a way that Lucy can answer. You know, she just gets the plot.

The thing I love is that the expectations are high. They expect Lucy to just jump in there and do it with all the other kids; they're not expecting her to be thick, and so she ain't thick.

They've got funding for her to have support and she does all the same classes, but hers is just that lower level, it's them sort of tempering it down to be manageable for her. Maths, they've got this book called Year Eight Maths, and Lucy's doing what is called Year Five, but it's the same book, it looks the same, and she's doing bits with that. They sort of try and modify things.

As long as Lucy is progressing and learning in class, that's what we want, and she gets all the other benefits that go with it. She's with the other kids. Then there are things like music and dance, well she can just do it with everyone else. So she's loving that ...

She has had an invitation, which I was thrilled to bits about, because she never got one at primary school. These girls asked her if she'd like to go out shopping to Harbour Town, there were four girls, they went together, they were all happy, though I don't know whether they'll contact her again.

We're having a bad patch at the moment, where she doesn't seem to want to go, but up until now she'd say, 'I love it.' I think she loves the stimulation, she loves being with all these other kids.

At the time I spoke to them both, Lucy certainly had nothing negative to say about school at all: she liked it, she liked her new friends, and though she didn't have a big group of friends to hang out with, she was able to 'pick some friends out and talk to them.' As a year eight student, she said she had lots of different subjects, too many to name, and she liked all of them, though cooking appeared to be a particular favourite. She had understandably found the new high school 'a bit scary' after her small Catholic primary school. When I asked her about catching the bus to school she said, 'The first time I started I was a bit scared, but now I've got the hang of it, it's fine.' Overall Lucy is, as her mother said, a pioneering type who will have a go and make the most of a new situation. She wants to be a journalist when she finishes school and is prepared to do the extra study to make it happen.

Rebecca Innes was less enthusiastic about her years of schooling in a mainstream setting. Rebecca spent kindergarten to year twelve in the inclusive setting of a small independent Anglican school in a town south of Perth. With her mother's support and a lot of intensive tuition at home, she graduated as an articulate and well-spoken young woman who subsequently undertook a traineeship at the local council, further study at TAFE and, later, study at university level in creative writing. As a recently graduated eighteen year old in 2006 however, her recollections of her school years were not favourable.

Jan: Did you enjoy school?

Rebecca: No, I didn't.

Jan: Tell me more

Rebecca: Well I didn't, no. I want to get school out of my mind. I went through, kindergarten to high school, I had a long period in school and I wanted to get it all done with. I went through high school, I went to year twelve, I graduated in year twelve and that was it, I was in the future.

When I interviewed her again three years later, Rebecca was more forthcoming.

Rebecca: It doesn't really affect me, but at school they never ever thought I was bright enough to do school, because nobody in the world could help anyone with Down syndrome. It was hard for them to help me. To me, Jan, I liked pre-primary school and kindergarten and primary the best. I didn't like high school ever. I didn't like high school.

Jan: Why was that?

Rebecca: I had friends in kindergarten and also friends in pre-primary, but in high school I didn't have any friends at all, Jan.

Jan: Why do you think that was?

Rebecca: Because they were just spoiling me, teasing me, kicking, going through my locker. They did all nasty things to me and they were kind of taking advantage of my disability. I didn't like that at all.

Jan: Did you know any other kids with disabilities at school?

Rebecca: No, I didn't. No one in high school, Jan, no one had Down syndrome there. I was the only child who had Down syndrome. Everyone just picked on me because I was different, because people who are different, normal kids can pick on people who are different. I didn't like it at all Jan. My life was horrible. I just don't want the same thing happening to other people.

Like Rebecca Innes, Alex Major also recalled being bullied at school, though overall he said he loved his time in the education support unit at a private boys school in Perth; and as for the bullying, he took steps to stop it.

Alex: I remember the mongrel moments, where I brought a gun to school once.

Jan: A gun, a real gun?

Alex: Plastic. It was about twice. I'd been caught by the cops just outside the school.

Jan: Did it look like a real gun?

Alex: Yes. Genuine.

Jan: What did they say?

Alex: Nothing, just, take the gun home and never do it. But the next day I brought a knife and tried to threaten someone with it. A Swiss Army knife.

Jan: Why did you take these weapons to school?

Alex: I don't know. I wanted to be safe. Bullies were picking on me, they were calling me names and telling me what to do. Yes, telling me to steal other people's lunches.

Jan: Did you tell the teachers about this?

Alex: Yes, I did tell the education support officer at our school, yes. They were in mainstream. They were year twelve at the time. I was younger. I would have been in year nine, ten. After that they stopped picking on me.

Jan: Did they bully everybody, or just pick on you?

Alex: Picked on me mainly, because I was only a kid then.

Alex now has a brown belt in tae kwon do.

Jeremy Young also recalled being bullied at school by another student with a disability, and fear of bullying haunted other parents such as Loretta Muller, as their children approached high school.

> I worry that the social side of things will not be very nice. That is probably the biggest thing that I worry about. That he will get teased or bullied or just not have very nice experiences. I had a really rough time at high school myself being badly bullied and I just don't want any of my kids to have that and especially him because he is going to be even more defenceless than anybody else.

The physical safety of their children was a concern for parents. Though any child can get lost, this seems to be a particular problem for children with Down syndrome as some have a heightened propensity to wander off. Though it makes a good story later in life, at the time such behaviour is potentially serious and desperately worrying for parents. Alex Major was delighted to describe how at his primary school he was always referred to as 'the great escape artist' because he constantly ran away.

> **Alex**: Well I decided to dig a little tunnel under some bushes in the corner of a courtyard, and from there I started escaping from that.
>
> **Jan**: Did you do that more than once, escape more than once?

Alex: Yes. One time they caught me at the beach, swimming. Naked! And the second time I got caught down at the train lines.

Train tracks also featured in Trish Weston's decision to take her son Will out of one particular school because of its derelict attitude to his safety.

We went along for an interview with the principal of the ed. support centre and voiced our concerns that we had about Will being there, in that he was a terrible wanderer, well, a bolter, really; he was off like a flash if you turned your back. And the school was not fenced and one of the boundaries was a railway line and the others were busy roads and this was a huge worry to us. But we were reassured that they'd make sure that he was safe there.

So off he went to the ed. support centre and proceeded to run away virtually every day that he was there and, in fact, on one awful occasion, actually was on the railway line, and I guess probably the worst thing about it was that a member of the public found him up on the level crossing and took him back to school and, in fact, they hadn't even noticed that he was missing, so that was a terrible worry for us and very stressful. So I thought, well, he'd already been lost a few times by then. I thought, well that will make them open their eyes a bit; but no, sure enough, he was off every opportunity he got. It's good to be able to laugh about it now but it really was a dreadful time!

Other parents have arrived unannounced at school to find their children unsupervised in the playground or pursuing their own activities entirely, instead of in class. Trish also recalled that particular experience.

When Will started at preschool there was a relief teacher who, to be quite frank, really didn't want Will to be there, and the feedback that we got from her was always negative. I don't know if he ever did do anything good, but certainly, if he did, we didn't hear about it, and he wasn't made to sit at mat time and he wasn't made to do the things that the other kids were doing, so he just ran riot and he'd take off outside and I didn't know about this until I turned up one day and found him out in the yard, which fortunately was securely fenced, pushing a doll's pram around the little pathway. And I went in and all the other children were doing various activities. And I said, 'Why is Will outside?' 'Oh well, he always does that when we are doing this.' And I said, 'Not any more!'

A reluctance on a teacher's part to discipline a child with a disability; the unhelpful 'dear little thing' attitude which leads to children getting away with normally unacceptable behaviour in the classroom: these practices very quickly teach children that they are not quite like the other kids and can do what their peers cannot. Equally, the child's peers learn the same thing. People who don't have a child with a disability will often tell you that children are blind to difference but most parents of a child with a disability know this is nonsense. Acceptance of second-rate behaviour or indeed any form of differential treatment identifies a child as 'different' and gives other children leave to regard them as such, inevitably leading to second-class status within the classroom.

In Rebecca's case she attributed her unhappiness at school less to the bullying than to her lack of friends.

My mum was trying to get someone to talk to the principal. My mum wanted some feedback, but she didn't get any feedback from school. I was in so much in pain at high school. I liked kindergarten, I liked pre-primary. Most of those friends Jan, just left. Most of my friends have left to different schools. When I walked into high school it was a completely different world altogether.

Fourteen year old Catherine Franklin would doubtless have agreed with Rebecca about the importance of friendship. She had friends, but they weren't her peers.

Catherine is always talking about friends. But she always makes friends with the older kids. She sits and has lunch with the year twelves or the year elevens and she is year nine. She doesn't seem to have much empathy with the kids her own age. And I think that is because she knows that she is not like them. I don't think she would articulate that, but she has got older siblings so she probably feels more comfortable with the kids who are older, who maybe don't expect as much of her. (Pamela Franklin)

Mark Brookton's parents were similarly concerned about his upper primary school playground routine.

They have a teacher on duty at recess and lunch and Mark's been hanging around with the teacher rather than going and playing. I don't want that. It's easier for him, because they talk and they respond, whereas he needs to be encouraged and they need to encourage him to be playing with his peers, not hanging around. (Wendy Brookton)

Rebecca's mother Penny was less negative than Rebecca about her school experience but agreed it had not always been ideal, particularly in the later years. The idea of fully inclusive schooling had motivated Penny from soon after Rebecca was born and, in what had initially been a very supportive school environment, this had originally been very successful. Penny recalled that when Rebecca had started school in the early 1990s, when she was about five, they had settled on a newly opening local private school because she thought the small school with a Christian focus would be a nurturing environment for her daughter. And indeed, Rebecca was welcomed.

I spoke to the headmistress before the school started and said, 'My daughter's got Down syndrome.' 'Oh, any child can come.' The school grew and Rebecca went right through from pre-primary right to year twelve.

It was great for the first probably five years and she had lots of friends and went to parties and things. Then the social life, the joining in — I think maybe year five, year six, when girls start getting catty — it sort of began petering out. I tried. I went to the school and talked about making friends and things. 'Oh well we can't make them be friends,' they said. 'Well that's not the idea,' I said, 'It's just kind of setting up a situation where she can have friends,' but they weren't willing to do it.

Other parents similarly felt the schools their children attended could have created an atmosphere which was more conducive to socialisation. Claudia Mansour, though she had liked many aspects of the co-ed Catholic college Theresa attended, believed the school had not gone very far in encouraging social interaction between children in the education support unit and mainstream students.

She hasn't been mistreated or teased, but she was never part of the other kids of the school. They could have encouraged, they could have circulated something. Living within the

Christian ethos which we have, we are all equal in the eyes of God and we all have our disabilities, all of us. Those kids have got it *showing*, we have got it hidden, and yes, I think that more could have been done.

Luke Middleton's daughter Laura attended a small independent school from the age of four, where she thrived on the system of supported full inclusion she enjoyed in the junior classroom; but her happiness didn't last as she progressed up the school. When Luke raised the question of Laura's increasing social isolation, one of the teachers told him that Laura 'had some issues to deal with as well.'

That hadn't occurred to me I must say. I thought it was the other kids' fault, not Laura's! She was right though, so we put a lot of time into making Laura more sociable: you know, getting her to look at people when she spoke to them; getting her to say 'hello' to people when they spoke to her; getting her to respond; getting her to initiate conversations; trying to get her to engage in conversations with people, with kids, but still the kids continued to drop off, when they got more cliquey and when they developed faster than she did, and Laura wasn't interested in their interests. That kind of thing ...

Certainly as kids with Down syndrome get older, they sometimes appear to reject gestures of friendship because of socially unskilled or inappropriate responses, which can be read as a lack of interest in socialising with their peers. Pamela Franklin however believed there was more to it than this.

At lunchtime last year Catherine used to wander around sort of talking to herself and some of the kids would say, 'Come and sit with us,' or whatever and she would always say no.

But I mean, I put myself in her place, if she goes and sits down with these kids, she is going to think she has to join in the conversation. What is she actually going to say that is going to be meaningful? And the kids are talking about things that she probably doesn't even understand in lots of ways. So, what she does is she compensates by performing and acting a bit stupid.

Laura's parents became increasingly dissatisfied with her school, 'not with the education necessarily because she was still developing quite quickly, but with what the school wasn't doing for inclusion.'

Across the years she lost all her friends at the school to the point where when her best friend, who also had Down syndrome, left she was more or less friendless there for two years. We tried to push the school for enhanced classroom inclusion, because we thought the problem started in the classroom and could be resolved there too, but neither the school nor the other parents with kids with disabilities were at all interested. (Luke Middleton)

Karen Langley was very impressed with most aspects of the same school, especially the education support staff, and believed it to be one of the best around for kids with disabilities. However, Karen's daughter Shannon had started school in the UK in an Oxbridge setting, where Karen thought she had probably experienced some of the best support and inclusion practices in the world, and consequently, like Laura's family, she saw concrete opportunities for improvement in their new school in Western Australia.

And it would not actually have taken that much effort on their part to make it exemplary. But you have to have the will to do so, and I understand as well that that is guided, especially in private schools, by the people who are paying the fees; and as it turned out, of about nine or ten families of children with special needs in the school, there were only two who were interested in changing things at all. And, in fact, the whole process served to alienate our two families from the others, because they all felt that we were undermining the excellent support that was already provided at the school. While we felt that things could be improved enormously, most of the families who have children with special needs in that school felt they were very lucky to have got them there and would do anything rather than have things changed, I think.

For Rebecca and Penny Innes, the crunch really came once Rebecca finished her primary schooling. Though Penny was concerned about the fall off in social opportunities, she was equally focused on Rebecca's academic progress.

The headmistress who had been so *for* Rebecca had left by that time and it had all changed. In fact I'd said to her in about year six that I didn't know whether this was the right school for Rebecca for when we go to high school, it's so academic. She said, 'No, we'll have a program, we'll set it up so that it works well for Rebecca.' Of course then she left, and after that their ethos was not to take in any more children with disabilities. So there were one or two kids who were remedial, but that was all. I'd find teachers who really wanted to help and then other teachers who'd just say, 'Well if she can't keep up, she can't keep up, mate,' you know. Then it became difficult.

I did look at a few other avenues, but I still felt that was the right school at the time. Then it came to round year ten, it was becoming even more academic. They were more interested in their results than the kids, I felt.

Penny and Rebecca tried a number of other alternatives at that time, including a vocational education and training (VET) program at the local high school but eventually they recommitted to her existing school though with increasingly limited optimism.

I must admit those two years, the year getting ready for year eleven and then year eleven, I was in tears half the time for the way they were treating her.

However, Penny had a parallel strategy in place for Rebecca. Through a local organisation dedicated to inclusive education for kids with disabilities, Rebecca accessed an intensive series of reading and numeracy programs which she used at home throughout her school years. In many respects the learning strategies Rebecca developed through these programs were more rigorous than those she acquired at school. The programs were premised on the belief that, given appropriate support, people with disabilities could certainly learn — and sometimes they learnt in spite of their school-based education. And they started young.

Reading, well I don't know what I really thought, but the point is that you get a child to read before they go to school, so that when they go to school the teachers can see that our children are educable. So that's what we did ...

Rebecca and another little girl of the same age, with cerebral palsy, worked together even before preschool, then all the way through preschool and by the time she was going into year one, she was just about reading[95] ...

We maintained reading and numeracy programs all the way through. I stopped a couple of times thinking that she's doing lots at school, but we would monitor her and she'd drop down when she wasn't doing the programs. We did stop for a while at high school because there was so much homework. Then after a while I said, 'I think this is more important than what she's doing at school, so we went back onto it and she hasn't really dropped back. (Penny Innes)

Certainly home education — offering their children additional educational programs in tandem to sending them off to school — was a priority for a number of the families interviewed, including mine. Iris Fisher used direct instruction programs for reading and literacy with her granddaughter Trudy for as long as she could.

I used to work through the various DISTAR books with language, reading and maths.[96] Yes, by myself. See, I didn't get in until late doing this work with Trudy, because I didn't know that they could be taught like this. I didn't know their capabilities. All those years I wasted. And after school, it may be only ten minutes a night, sometimes half an hour. Weekends, I used to perhaps spend half an hour to an hour or more a day; and during these years, Trudy herself would vary as to how good she was. In a good period, which might run many months, I would just work through the programs bang, bang, bang. Other times, she would almost forget everything she'd ever learnt and these periods might go for one, two months. And it didn't matter, I could go back to the first book, the first page. And sometimes I could get her not remembering anything, but then suddenly she would come back to where she'd been before, and it was not till down the track that I realised that the inconsistencies probably were all medical.

The Brooktons in the far north of the state had been involved with the same parent educational group used by Penny and Rebecca Innes from the time Mark (born 1993) was about four. The programs had been far more than just a backstop — at one stage, when Mark was expelled from his local Catholic school and was home-schooled for six months, they were his educational lifeline. Living nearly 4000 kilometres from the group's base presented its own challenges but video enabled the program to work.

> We were the first people ever to have done all our teaching training by video. We only met the program's director about four years after we'd been teaching. (Wendy Brookton)

Wendy Brookton was adamant about the importance of the group's educational support to their lives as well as Mark's. It was invaluable in terms of Mark's education by accelerating his learning in a number of critical areas, and given the family concrete teaching skills, but it had also taught them strategies for dealing with the system as a whole.

> What did we get? Hope probably. That there was someone out there that could really relate to where we were at, that we wanted to help our child, and that we were in the best position to help our child. As parents. We needed to take control. That was probably the biggest thing that we learned, that if we don't take control, no one else is going to have the same input into Mark's life as we will.

Living in the far north, the Brooktons and other families like them had few educational options. Sandra Rossi went to the local high school and experienced no particular difficulties, but for her family, her long-term medical treatment was of far greater concern. Frank Flynn went south with his mother where he attended Millen special school in Perth, the same school Geoffrey Mann attended; but that was the beginning of the severing of the links with his local Kimberley community. Charlie King attended the local Catholic school where his mother and sister both taught till he was in his late teens, though it was only a primary school. There was no secondary school in their town, and his sister Marg, who herself went down south to school, endorsed her mother's decision to keep Charlie local for schooling.

> I used to believe, sending your children away, they get a better education. Yeah, for some people it works, but there's a lot who likes family.

In both Frank's and Charlie's cases, the educational decisions their families made had a big impact in later years in terms of their continuing relationships with their Aboriginal families and communities, discussed in later chapters.

The experiences of families in the far north unfortunately reinforce the point made by the Department of Education in Western Australia to a Senate inquiry in 2002.

> The provision of services to small populations, and often individual students with high needs, presents significant resourcing and operational challenges ... These challenges are shared by other Government agencies involved in supporting students with disabilities. They may result in less available, less sophisticated and reliable support. Special programs which require a critical mass of students and high level employee skills ... may prove practically impossible to establish and maintain in rural and remote areas even if there were no significant funding constraints.[97]

Nearly a decade later, the situation is little better.

For people with Down syndrome, as for all children, school years can range from depressing to wonderful. For parents though, education is undoubtedly a minefield. The shift from the earliest approach entailing no more than training people with intellectual disabilities such as Down syndrome in special segregated institutions, through the development of special education centres and units, to integration and mainstreaming and ultimately to full inclusion, is a process which has been driven by both parents and advocates but it is not without its critics. The Australian government's 2002 Senate inquiry into education reported that

> inclusive education ... is widely accepted as likely to lead to the most desirable learning outcome for students. Inclusive education also recognises the human rights and equal entitlements of those with disabilities and embraces certain social responsibilities and ethical goals which are supposed to be consistent with a polity such as Australia. [However] there is considerable evidence that some of these responsibilities are proving to be onerous.[98]

As this chapter has shown, both children and parents can become casualties in ideological wars about education, with the school as the battleground. What seems like inclusion on the outside might look more like token mainstreaming on the inside. Finely tuned inclusion programs which have been supported by parents and teachers have failed for individual children. Other children in a variety of settings have sailed happily through their educational years with far less monitoring and intervention.

As parents we found ourselves at times receiving flak from both sides of the 'inclusion' divide. At our daughter's primary school we were accused of being 'in denial' — a phrase usually thrown at parents who find themselves unable to face up to the reality of having a child with a disability — when we and another family pushed for a more inclusive environment for our children. The other family subsequently withdrew their daughter from the school. And we ourselves were later asked to leave an inclusive education organisation after we enrolled our daughter in the high school of her choice (the special education unit of the Catholic college where her friends were already enrolled), because our actions were at odds with the organisation's ethos of total commitment to educational inclusion. For us, the unacceptable price of the total educational inclusion the group advocated was the loss of Maddie's existing social network. They intimated we weren't prepared to go the distance. As the solution they offered to us entailed a twice daily fifty-kilometre round trip across the city to the nearest inclusive environment the group would endorse, with likely damage to our daughter's existing friendships and severe disruption to our other two daughters' social lives and our own working lives, they were right. But we also lost access to their invaluable educational programs.

Like some other parents, we also fought personal demons over Maddie's high school enrolment. Though she was extremely happy there, we agonised every one of her high school years over whether the school we had opted for was the best choice either educationally or socially, and enrolling her there was certainly at odds with our own philosophical belief in inclusion. Though inclusion seemed to be working admirably for Lucy Burton, her mother Heather recognised that her own commitment to inclusion sprang from her personal reluctance to deal with the implications of a supported educational environment. Britt Canning and Virginia Robb both shifted from their preferred position of full inclusion to a much less inclusive setting for the sake of their children's happiness. Karen Langley ultimately pulled her daughter Shannon out of a small local high school and placed her in a specialist school for students with disabilities where her growth in self-confidence and self-esteem has been enormous.

Inclusion is not the only issue. Access to educational choices is also dependent on location. There are fewer choices in the country, where attending the local government school with minimal support is sometimes the standard practice outside the metropolitan areas. While this may compromise educational outcomes, going to school in a smaller town can also foster social inclusion. How does one balance educational gains against social gains? Why have many parents found it so hard to attain both?

Not every parent wants educational inclusion for their child. Those who do, however, generally view educational inclusion as part of a process of social inclusion which relates to all marginalised groups within society; one cannot work properly without the other.

> I still believe that the more 'normal' the setting you can create for this child, the more 'normal' things are going to end up, on both sides. I mean, both in terms of the child with special needs and also in society at large. If all those kids in Shannon's class had grown up through their years in school with this child with Down syndrome as one of the group and had learnt to understand her with her speech impediment and to take account of her differences, and even help her out if she needs a bit of help, they would have a totally different attitude than a kid like me, for example, who had never spoken to anyone else with Down syndrome until long after Shannon was born. So I think that it is really important that inclusion happens and goes ahead. And, given that education is a huge social thing for kids at this age as well, I think it's probably the main area to be focusing on. (Karen Langley)

Where full inclusion is absent from society as a whole though, it is hardly surprising that you can't always find it in the classroom.

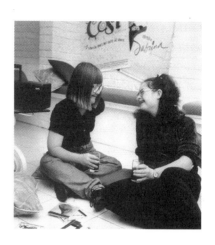

chapter 6

SCHOOL'S OUT:
THE RIGHT AND RITES OF PASSAGE

The transition to adult life can be a challenging one for people with disabilities and their families. From the ultimately reasonably comfortable and familiar vantage point of the school years, the future can appear confronting, representing as it does the end of childhood. Entering the workforce is a milestone many parents of people with disabilities anticipate with trepidation. Recreation needs can also become more demanding once school no longer fills a young person's days and by this stage too, parents find that issues associated with independence and adulthood — such as relationships and sexuality, issues they might prefer to ignore — must be addressed.

When a teenager with a disability turns sixteen, they become eligible to apply for the Commonwealth government's Disability Support Pension which, for most people with Down syndrome, is likely to remain their chief source of income indefinitely. The year before they leave school, they can also apply for post school options (PSO) funding, which is part of the Western Australian state government's Alternatives to Employment (ATE) program to assist people with disabilities who are not able to work full-time to access support for recreational and similar activities.[99]

Like the pension, the needs-based ATE support is not guaranteed. For the parents, applying for ATE necessitates the sometimes difficult task of reassessing their child's capacities and skills. The process includes a rigorous series of forms and interviews which serve to tease out a child's weak points. It is a painful procedure and for many parents, having become accustomed for years to celebrating the positive aspects of their child's achievements, it can feel like a real betrayal of that child and their values. Yet the reality is, particularly for people with disabilities not able to undertake full-time work and perhaps unlikely to earn more than a minimal salary in supported employment, additional financial support is essential. The availability of ATE or other forms of funding such as Intensive Family Support can mean the difference between a relatively full and active life and one spent sitting at home. And as some parents realise very starkly once their family member with a disability leaves school, the way they fill their day can impact not just on the individual but the entire family.

There is plenty of room for optimism. The pathways available for a young person with a disability are similar to those available to other school leavers. Most people with Down syndrome pursue a combination of employment, social, recreational, study and volunteer activities. Opportunities sometimes come faster than expected and many parents felt that the transition from school was actually much less daunting than they had anticipated.

There is no 'typical' way of using ATE funding; where it is allocated, it can be used in a range of ways to suit the needs of the individual, and might include personal or group recreation support (paying for a support worker to accompany you swimming or to a movie, for instance), assistance in a study environment or transport training. Will Weston (born 1984) receives ATE funding which gives him around twelve to fourteen hours of recreational activities a week, complementing his three days a week gardening and outdoor maintenance employment through an agency, in a small team of three young men with disabilities and a supervisor. His was a smooth transition to the workplace.

> He really sees himself as a working man now, not a school kid. It's a joy to see him going to work three days a week — keen to go — at 7.30 a.m.! He also loves his ATE days and looks forward to the social and recreational activities. He has other inclusive sports on the weekend which he is passionate about. He has a great life really — I worried a lot about him leaving school but I shouldn't have. (Trish Weston)

Access to meaningful employment for people with intellectual disabilities, like access to education, is a legacy of the parent groups which advocated from the 1950s for their children to be recognised as citizens. Educational facilities emerged in the context of postwar negotiation over the meaning of disability and the rights of the disabled, but as historian Charlie Fox observed, 'It didn't take long for the [parent] associations to realise that once their children had finished school that there was nowhere else for them to go.'[100] In the early 1950s members of the SLCG began to advocate the purchase of farms to become 'colonies' where children and young adults could be trained and employed and live safely and permanently once their parents died.[101] At the same time, the notion of training for those who could live more independently gained currency in SLCG circles, with manual training and gardening advocated for the boys and domestic work and mothercraft for girls.[102] Training was viewed as a step towards independence and, for girls, was deemed 'essential for their own home in the future and also maybe the means of employment.'[103]

Training programs for independent employment did not materialise at that stage, but employment itself did. The SLCG opened their own 'sheltered workshops' from the 1950s and within decades they had grown into the multi-million dollar business which is Activ Industries today. In Activ's early days as SLCG, a large proportion of the employees had Down syndrome.[104] Today, Activ employs more than one thousand men and women across the metropolitan area and in regional Western Australia in supported employment workplaces (now more usually referred to as disability enterprises) dealing with textiles, timber products, metal products, property care, packaging and assembly and print finishing. Beyond disability enterprises, Activ Foundation also provides a raft of recreation, social and travel opportunities for its members and clients.

Sheltered workshops were the first employment opportunities made available for people with intellectual disabilities once they moved out of institutions and into the community; previously, if they had worked at all, their workplace was also their home. From the late 1960s the federal government began to fund sheltered employment but there was little if any attempt to breach the walls of sheltered workshops and move workers with disabilities into community workplaces. Not only prospective employers, but parents and workshop personnel themselves were largely pessimistic or dismissive of the prospect of employment outside workshops.[105] This remained the situation in Western Australia until the 1980s when the possibility of supporting employees with disabilities in open (mainstream) employment in the community was mooted more seriously. Employment support agencies such as we know today gradually emerged, with a new focus on matching individuals to suitable open employment positions and working intensively on a one-on-one basis, training individual workers on the job until both worker and employer were happy that the job had been mastered — though ongoing employment support is seldom if ever withdrawn entirely.

Across Western Australia today there are nearly one hundred Australian-government funded employment agencies with the broad brief of supporting people with a spectrum of physical, cognitive, intellectual and psychiatric disabilities in both open and 'supported' employment. Of approximately 7800 Western Australians (9.4 per cent of the national total) across the range of disabilities and conditions using these services in 2006–07, about 70 per cent were in open employment and 30 per cent in supported employment services. There appears to be no accessible data on the number of people with Down syndrome using these services, but going on figures in the most recent government Disability Services Census (2008), in 2006–07, 58 per cent of all people with intellectual disability using employment support services nationally were in supported employment (or disability enterprises), with the remainder in open employment. This indicated a slight shift towards supported employment from open employment since 2000–01, when just under half (47 per cent) were in open employment and slightly more (53 per cent) in supported employment.[106] These figures may give some indication of the situation for people with Down syndrome in Western Australia.

Trevor Simpson and Geoffrey Mann have both spent decades in the supportive and familiar environment of disability enterprises such as Activ Industries. Straight after he finished school in the late 1950s, Trevor (born 1943) took up employment at one of the earliest of the SLCG workshops. This was the forerunner to the Osborne Park workshop and for Trevor, it involved packing newspapers, but he later moved on to more skilled work.

> He's mainly in the metal workshop now and he can operate various machines, but they tend to change the jobs very often and I think he doesn't like change too much, you see, and he's missed out on learning a few new things because he likes to stay where he is. The work varies, and sometimes they don't have any work at all, so they find various occupations. He might be watching a video or anything. I don't know exactly how often that happens but Trevor is happy there. He's not interested in going anywhere else. Some of his friends have moved on to other workshops, but he always says no, he doesn't want to go anywhere else. He wants to stay with his friends. There are quite a lot who are his age and older, I think, and it's just unfortunate that the chances of outside employment or even more employment in the workshop are not there. And some of the ideas for getting them into open employment I think are quite unrealistic. However, it depends on the individual. (Mavis Simpson)

Geoffrey Mann (born 1967) left school at the age of sixteen and like Trevor, took up a position in a SLCG workshop. His parents had put his name down for a vacancy some time previously and had not anticipated him being offered the sought-after placement before he turned eighteen, the school leaving age, but when the offer came unexpectedly in the early 1980s they were reluctant to let the opportunity pass.

> Although the workshop was able to offer him industrial packaging or working in the nursery, he was very clear in his mind that woodwork was his only interest, and he still is a confirmed woodwork man. At first all the work he did was sweeping up the shavings from the floor and sanding, hand sanding timber endlessly for hours and hours. And when the parent group suggested that maybe we could raise money and buy the workshop a sander, a sanding machine, we were told that if we did, there'd be nothing to give the severely disabled to do. However, things have been changed very much since those days. The workshop is now lined with quite sophisticated woodworking machinery and Geoffrey and most of the boys who work in that section are now multi-skilled, in the current jargon. They've been taught to operate all these machines, including sanding machines, drills and various other things. So he has learnt as he's gone along there, and the standard of their products is really amazing, it's very impressive. It used to be mainly jarrah garden furniture, outdoor furniture, but now Geoffrey's particular workshop has swung to occasional indoor furniture, like coffee tables and telephone tables, nests of tables and planter boxes and they are really attractive items of furniture. The boys take a great pride in what's produced. (Muriel Mann)

Like Trevor's mother, Geoffrey's parents were very positive about his experiences in the closed environment of the workshop, though his father had some worries about the future.

After we're dead he might be pushed into open employment and because he has experience with timber, perhaps put into a place where there's a much wider range of equipment than he's been trained to use, and he'll get what people call the shit work and have to sweep the floor and do the sanding and go and fetch the lunches, whereas now he builds things and there's a certain degree of pride. I took Geoffrey to the Royal Show a couple of years ago and we went into the furniture display and there was a beautiful desk and Geoffrey walked up to that desk and looked at it and ran his hand over the surface. Now that's the sort of thing a craftsman does, and I thought, 'My God, he's really learning something!' (William Mann)

The average age of employees in supported industries such as Activ is higher than in open employment but for younger people too, as the statistics show, open employment is not always the first choice. Issues such as social inclusion, dignity, self-confidence and friendship require fine-tuning and sometimes trade-offs to achieve the appropriate balance for each individual but, as in the educational sphere, at least now there are some alternatives.

The obvious benefits of providing people with intellectual disabilities with work is that it gives their life structure, meaning and direction, while for employers, the benefits have included a dedicated and responsible workforce, and for the government and the state, it means citizens in productive work. Purely on a cost basis, facilitating open employment and disability enterprises helps reduce the government's payout on disability pensions, though a government disability pension still remains the chief source of income for most people in supported employment.[107] This is not surprising considering that in supported employment in Western Australia in 2006–07, the majority of people worked part time, the average gross hourly rate of pay was $2.26 and the average gross weekly wage was $59.83.[108] However, the pay is not necessarily the most important thing, as Steph Webb said after her daughter Nicola found a job in open employment.

> It's not so much being paid for the job, it's getting out there and doing something. I'd even pay someone to employ her, just to get out there and be part of the community instead of just sitting at home all the time.

When Angus Grant (born 1971) finished school in his late teens, he went to a farm school in the northern Perth suburb of Landsdale for a while before starting work through Activ Industries. That was not particularly successful; his family was told he was disruptive, though his father Bernard was more inclined to think problems were caused by a personality clash. Nonetheless he was left unemployed and, worse, unoccupied, an experience Bernard described as 'dreadful' for both Angus and his family. Eventually however, he found a place working with electronic assembly where he got on 'like a house on fire'.

> That was an interesting place because it wasn't a sheltered workshop as such; it was a mix of so-called normal and disabled people. But a very family atmosphere type small workshop. He had his troubles from time to time, but basically did quite well. He's very, very good at repetitive things, as long as you keep his nose to the wheel. He must have been there about ten years, pretty much full time, which was great. He was getting $20 a week I think, for full-time work, but that wasn't the point for us. It proved that when he was provided with the proper supervision, Angus could hold his own in the workforce.

Then the firm closed down and the workers were transferred to another workshop at Bassendean. However, when he was in his late twenties, he was hospitalised for some weeks and when he came back they cut his hours to two and a half days a week. There was no consultation about that, and they haven't reinstated it, so he went from about thirty-five hours a week to sixteen and that's made a massive change. I really think he could work a thirty-five hour week. Maybe he doesn't need to. But that's not the purpose of the thing.

Angus now pursues a mix of work and recreational activities Monday to Friday but his parents' preference would have been for him to remain more fully involved with 'work that was meaningful.'

In Perth, government-funded employment agencies are available to help job seekers who want open employment. They find positions appropriate to their skills, and they can negotiate with the employer to ensure the person and the position are a good match. Wages are usually paid on the basis of an agreed formula according to the person's productivity on the job. Finding the right placement is not always a quick process, and sometimes there's a bit of luck involved, but the results can often last long term. When she left school, Theresa Mansour (born 1976) contacted an employment agency to assist her in finding open employment. Their first step was to provide her with transport training to help her access different workplaces, but after half a year of retail and hospitality work experience in businesses such as Hungry Jack's, Kmart and Target, she still didn't have a paid job. Theresa's personal preference was for office work so her mother, who was on the auxiliary of a local hospital, came up with her own solution. With the help of the employment agency, they approached the hospital.

They took Theresa on board and the social worker went with her a few times, helping her so she could master the job on her own. And the agency checks on her every month, they get feedback from her bosses and Theresa just fitted in. I can't believe it, the Lord has done all this, it's so wonderful, so close to home. Theresa has blossomed. I think she grew overnight, you know. The atmosphere, all her colleagues, all her friends there, they're absolutely wonderful ...

She works in the accounts department, she puts the envelopes in postcode order. She does the patients' wristbands. She sometimes does things for the postal department. She says, 'Today I am busy, I have a lot of things to do.' She stays back if she needs to. We told her, 'When you are busy, stay, finish your work.' (Claudia Mansour)

Theresa works five days a week and is paid for two hours daily at the normal rate but usually works from 8.30 till 11.30 to enable her to complete her work without stress. In addition she still gets some funding, though reduced, from a disability pension. Theresa started at the hospital at the age of nineteen and was still there in her thirties. As her mother said, 'She loves it. She loves the place. She can live there.'

Jeremy Young has also worked for years in open employment, in a government organisation where he is supported by an employment agency.

I work in West Perth. I like it there. Before I started in West Perth, I worked in Fremantle at the beginning and then Cannington.

When I first got the job I was doing work experience at the time — this was in 1992 — and finally they gave me the job, which was good. I felt very, very, very pleased about that. So I started off in Fremantle, and I worked there for a while, you know, got to know the staff there, well, more like work colleagues and stuff, which is great, because work colleagues are good people too. And I did jobs for everyone, filling up photocopiers and how to work a photocopier if they have jams or anything. And then I was moved from Fremantle to Cannington, where I did the same job then as well …

I caught the 155 bus to Albany Highway, and then a small bus from Albany Highway. Anyway, just one long bus, one short bus, that got me in at nine, because my hours were nine to one-thirty. Five days a week. And it was stressful because of the long hours from getting up early, catching the bus, which took an hour each way, and I didn't really like it at all. And that was how I didn't see my life. And then two people came into my work in Cannington and asked if I could come down to West Perth, and I did. So I was transferred down there. And now I feel like I've been in West Perth all my life now. And it's less stressful, because I am now catching the train, and — same hours, from nine to one-thirty, and I do jobs, different jobs to the one I was doing in Cannington. Still filling up the photocopiers, and doing data now on computer, which I now have on my desk, which is great. I do data like government cars — you know, like car washings every Monday and going down to the cars and taking out log sheets and bringing them in. Like the miles and the kilometres they do, and the mail run every morning and all sorts of other different jobs too. Yes, I have three months long service leave now, and I am not quite sure how I am going to take them, because I'm trying to save. Still trying to get some Lottos to help me with that!

Jeremy subsequently moved to yet another location, at Myaree, still within the same organisation. Here his duties have included supervising a number of work experience students and trainees.

Outside Perth, lifestyle and life chances are very different. Charlie King (born 1965), an Aboriginal man from the Kimberley, is blessed with a big family of siblings and moves comfortably among them, from one home to another, as the mood takes him. Charlie left school at about seventeen and his sisters Marg King and Rhonda Henry recall that at that stage, there had been some talk of sending him away to a residential home for further training but his mother refused. She had been led to believe when he was a baby that he would not live much beyond his teen years, and 'this thing had played on her mind, so she nourished everything she could get out of him. But he's lived to forty; he's proven a lot of people wrong.'

After Charlie's mother died, his siblings and his extended family all took on his care and he does not access any government-funded employment or recreational support.

> For anyone with a disability, I really believe family support is the most important thing. For anyone without that family support, I think you'd be lost. You'd feel like nobody. We've pretty much got that feeling, keeping people together. (Marg King)

Charlie's extended 'family' encompasses more than most people's. His mother's and now his sisters' households are large ones and not confined to blood relations, with anyone who needed a bed or a feed always made welcome. The idea of reciprocity is strong and this network of family and friends has always kept a lookout for Charlie. Though he has never had a regular job Charlie helps out when and where it suits him.

Every now and then he'll go out with somebody he knows and just do whatever they're doing, make out he's working. When he was living in Lombadina with his uncles, they did rubbish truck, so they'd chuck him in with them. He doesn't do anything; he just sits there and gives the orders. He's the supervisor, and they just bring him along. It's like, you know, how a young child will go and work to earn a feed or earn ten dollars. Charlie would go over to the closest shop. And anyhow he ended up taking over the watering and sweeping for them. They'd pay him with a hamburger, maybe a packet of smokes and a cool drink, or whatever he wanted to eat. Mum didn't mind, she didn't think of it as cheap labour, she thought it was good, kept him busy. (Marg King and Rhonda Henry)

Charlie also likes to do some work with the local Shire, helping to clean up the road; he loves working at the rodeo and enjoys taking water to the cattle. His life is not structured the way it would probably be if he lived in a larger town or had more formal 'services' but it is safe, full and satisfying and is focused on the family and his community.

Also in the Kimberley, Mark Brookton was already well on the way to adult independence while still at high school. He rides horses, loves motocross and by the time he was twelve had already bought his own motorbike with money he had earned. His parents had never questioned his capacity to succeed and when Mark was just twelve, his father was confident of Mark's post school prospects.

Yes, I think the future's pretty good for Mark. I think the community's good for him too. Like he's got a job, he mows our lawn, he gets paid for that. Up the road he's got another job, he mows the lawn up there, so he's got two lawn mowing jobs. Just people in the community — he'll get a job. (Keith Brookton)

Just a few years later, Mark was organising his gardening as a small business, sending out accounts and managing his own finances.

Rachel Kingston (born 1980) works at Coles in the northern suburbs three hours a day, five days a week, and takes a bus to work from her shared apartment in Subiaco. She has been there over a decade and has a long service award. 'I go and show the customers all the aisles,' she said. 'I can help you find whatever you want.' Rachel is proud of her skills and very fond of her work colleagues, though she did experience teasing in the workplace at one stage, which her boss quickly put a stop to.

Rachel's flatmate Eloise Hartley, who is the same age, has worked part time for eight years at a sports goods outlet in West Perth, with the support of her employment agency. But she sees this as just one aspect of her life.

I hang up clothes. I tag shoes. Put price stickers on the socks and tops. I don't mind working there for a few years, but I'm actually working on my acting career now. I started acting in high school and I did a lot of theatre. Then I went on to DADAA.[109] That's when they had lots of festivals and workshops. So I picked drama. It was quite fun. I got to meet lots of people. I also went through the Academy, the Academy of Performing Arts [at Edith Cowan University]. I did a one-year course there. Yes I kind of studied with a lot of people. There was a group of people. Then we did some role-playing. You know, like skills.

Eloise was given an award by Variety Club for dedication to her acting and is presently working on a production in conjunction with a former school friend.

She's actually helping me do this one-woman play. I am going to play myself. It's going to be about my journey through life. I've been into film courses. We're getting more people to come in and work with me and get some more acting experience and skills and make me a better performer.

Alex Major (born 1982) combines work with study and in both spheres he has taken on responsible roles representing people with disabilities. He has two jobs. One day a week he works at a local bottle shop making up speciality beer and wine packs and another two days a week he works from 8.30 a.m. until 3.25 p.m. with Activ Industries in Osborne Park, where he has been employed for seven years. A number of parents and some young adults themselves were unenthusiastic about the prospect of working in a disability enterprise, with the old notion of a 'sheltered workshop' being only one step away from an institution, still very much part of the perception of how disability enterprises operate. Loretta Muller and Steph Webb for instance, both said they thought their kids were 'a bit better than that,' and Nicola Webb said she found the work in two different disability enterprises 'boring' and was much happier when she moved into open employment. Alex though is a young man who is holding down one job in open employment but at the same time has found real responsibility and personal agency in his other job in an Activ disability enterprise.

We work in teams. Every team has a leader and a general hand, a leading hand person. In my team the leading hand is me. And I'm on the committee there as well, as a committee member for the employees — that's us and some other people in the other teams — we see what's dangerous, assess the risk, make changes. I've been on that for three years now.

At his TAFE (Technical and Further Education) college, Alex is also on the student council.

Alex: If people are in trouble they come to me for help, like if people are harassing them, they come and see me as well.

Jan: Are these people with disabilities?

Alex: Yes. Learning disabilities, and other different disabilities as well.

Jan: How did you get that position?

Alex: There was an election. The main staff at Challenger TAFE, they nominated me to be a student leader, so I'm a student leader for the Council there.

Jan: You must be very proud.

Alex: I am actually.

Like Alex, many younger people with disabilities do further study at TAFE or at Institutes of Technology after leaving school, though Catherine Franklin (born 1984) began working towards TAFE qualifications while still at school; quite a few secondary schools offer students this option.

> The TAFE thing was really great because when she left school she was already there so it wasn't a big change. She was trained in terms of transport to get there and back with one of the teachers too. (Pamela Franklin)

TAFE offers a raft of choices designed for people with special learning needs, focusing on social and communication skills as well as academic and professional skills in areas such as retail, horticulture, business, hospitality and arts and design. Students with disabilities can also access regular courses. Offerings include a course in driver education, designed to get students to the point of passing their driver theory test before they commenced practical lessons. And the cost of the courses was, as Catherine's mother said, 'Ridiculous! It's something like $22 a year!' Catherine's nine-to-five life is certainly a very full one, with 'employment and volunteer work and TAFE —

that takes up four and a half days a week, so that's pretty good. She has Monday morning off.'

As well as part-time work and studying at TAFE, eighteen year old Laura Middleton has volunteered with Red Cross since leaving school.

> I go in to Fremantle Hospital on a Monday morning. First you have a coffee and then you start going through the wards. You go with someone else and we have a trolley with the magazines and you go in and ask the patients nicely if they would like a magazine. And you have to make sure you wash your hands every time you go in to a patient. There's a soap thing right near the door where you wash your hands. We start at half past nine and finish at half past eleven. I like talking to the other volunteer staff and I sometimes chat to the patients.

With support provided through her PSO (post school options) program, Laura is learning to travel independently to her work, study and recreational activities using public transport.

While still at school Rebecca Innes (born 1987) began hospitality education at the local Career Enterprise Centre, where she combined practical work with the TAFE course. As part of her post school options package she then undertook a 'learning for work' program and through her employment agency was subsequently offered a traineeship at the local council in the town south of Perth where she lived with her mother. The two-year program involved full-time work but also associated study. After six months Rebecca found it too much.

> Because I had long hours, I couldn't cope. My traineeship was hard. I ran through a health and safety thing and then

I couldn't do the homework. Like, I did work at work and then I did homework again when I got home and it was too much. So my supervisor cut down my hours so I do part time. It suits me a lot better.

For a while Rebecca remained part-time at the Council while studying complementary courses in computer skills at TAFE, but she eventually left to follow other employment avenues. After a series of different jobs, including working with younger children at a local primary school, she is now studying creative writing at Edith Cowan University.

There are some wonderful opportunities available for people with disabilities once they leave school, but not everyone is able to access or take advantage of them. Sometimes parents and children are faced with a future that doesn't look as promising as they might have hoped, though this is seldom a consequence of Down syndrome alone. Sandra Rossi, who lives in a regional town in the north-west, has health problems caused by dislocated hips as a child and an associated weight issue, which have made it virtually impossible for her to work 'because she can't stand for too long and she can't sit for too long.' Even pursuing recreational activities is a challenge.

A typical day she mainly gets up and potters around the house. I'll take her down the street, especially on her pay week I'll take her down and make her buy her toiletries and things, her videos. She gets her videos for the weekend and I make her walk the aisle without a wheelchair just to get the exercise and tire her out. She has a walking frame as well, but she doesn't like to use that very much. (Janet Rossi)

Her mother Janet's role as a carer is fundamental to Sandra's wellbeing and Janet reiterated what Charlie King's sisters said: 'Family members are your backbone support.' Sandra's sisters spend time with her and take her to their own homes at weekends. A family support agency, an organisation which Janet herself helped to develop in the region, also provides Sandra with recreation and Janet with important respite. But this is not always ideal, and friendship is a continuing issue.

The carer comes and she takes her for a drive, takes her down the beach, every second day. But with outsiders she has difficulty. I think over a period of time she's had a lot of carers, a lot of people in her life that didn't do the right thing by her. Not really acting in her interest, it was just a job to them sort of thing. Didn't have the patience with her. That affected her greatly where she got sick of people in and out of her life. When she developed a friendship with someone it wasn't a lasting friendship, they'd be off the scene after a short time because in this town finding carers is very hard and difficult, they're only here for like short term.

Now in her thirties, Sandra has accepted the direction of her life though, as her mother suggested, not completely happily. This is a source of continuing concern for her mother and family.

In the early stages, she used to express what she wanted to be and what she wanted to do and that, but I think she's now come to terms with what her life's like and she doesn't talk about it much. I mean she even used to go to the hotels and listen to a band because she loves music and things like that. She hasn't been doing that for a long time. I don't know, she's just becoming very reclusive of late, and we're trying to get her out of it. I think she's just lost her confidence because she's been off the scene for a long time.

As well as finding employment and daily occupation, there are other rites of passage associated with growing up and independence. Getting your driving licence is one. There may be less of an emphasis on this for people with Down syndrome, but many see their siblings and at least some of their peers learning to drive and often the desire for self-sufficiency is there. Quite a number of young people with Down syndrome do a driving course at TAFE, which is designed to teach students the road rules to an acceptable standard to pass the paper test, the first barrier towards gaining a full licence. For others, the barrier may be their parents, as twenty-five year old Nathan Johnson pointed out.

Nathan: I want to do a driving course some day.
Jan: Have you talked to your family about getting a licence?
Nathan: Yes.
Jan: What are their ideas?
Nathan: Well, Mum reckons driving is scary but I said I want to learn. That's one way of doing it. I want to get on with my life.
Jan: What did she say?
Nathan: Nervous!

Pamela Franklin was equally concerned about the prospect of her daughter Catherine driving.

Well she's going to do a driving course she reckons; but no, she'd be useless. Absolutely. I can imagine it — having to make decisions about a stop sign that's coming up and left turn only, or one-way street. I mean, some kids have done it. They can register to do this driving course at TAFE, but if they don't pass the initial thing well then they can't do it. So if she wants to do it I'm not going to stop her; if she keeps passing, she may as well keep going; but I can't see it happening myself.

Even where parents weren't too unhappy about the prospect of their teenager driving, there were sometimes other problems — which, for reluctant parents, could turn out to be a blessing. I asked Claudia Mansour whether she thought her daughter Theresa could learn to drive.

If her eyesight was good, I think so. Because she is very good with directions, she would know which way you had to go and where to go. But I really haven't thought much about it because I think that is a no-no because of her vision.

Attitudes seemed to be more flexible outside the metropolitan area. The Brooktons in the Kimberley both looked at me incredulously when I asked whether their son Mark would learn to drive. As the family lived twenty kilometres outside the nearest town, perhaps the answer was fairly obvious. 'Oh yes, have to!' How else was he going to get to work? In fact at the age of twelve, Mark was already driving the ute around the farm and his parents took a relaxed attitude, unfamiliar to most city parents, towards the whole process.

Keith: Having a farm's a lot easier too, because when they're learning to drive they hit a few things.
Wendy: Bounce off a few trees and things.
Keith: But it doesn't matter; they can go anywhere they like.

By the age of fifteen, Mark was working towards his boat licence.

Benita Diaz wanted to be like everyone else and driving a car was part of that. As a teenager she was desperately unhappy at her lack of height as she feared she might not be able to reach the car's pedals. She soon learned the road rules riding a bike, but her mother Ana thought she would not be able to go any further than that. However, she passed her written test at her first attempt. Next step was the practical and they found a driving school which offered lessons for people with disabilities, but at a fee ten dollars per hour more expensive than at a regular driving school.

> I said, 'Why?' He said, 'Oh yes, you know, we need more time.' I said, 'But you're coming for one hour!' My husband said, 'Forget it. You want her to do it?' and I said, 'I don't want her to do it, but she wants to do it, so okay.' So we gave her a chance. The first time they came, parking in the park bay. The second day, in the park. Oh yes, it was good, you know, she had to learn all the things — the brake, the handbrake, the steering wheel — but in the park. Third day still in the park, so I said, 'Thank you very much. Don't come any more. I can't afford it!'

Subsequently they found a teacher from a regular driving school at a regular price and Benita took two or three lessons a week, supplemented by practice sessions in the family car.

> The teacher said we need to help Benita sometimes with her driving, and I said, 'Okay, we'll give it a go.' Me, more than my husband, because my husband was very nervous. One day she stopped the car with him, got out of the car, came back home walking and said, 'I don't want to go any more with him!'

Benita had twelve months in which to pass her practical test, but she failed it twice.

And then the last week, I said, 'Benita, it's one year, no more. If you don't pass, you can't do it any more.' My husband said, 'Oh, she can go back again.' I said, 'I am not going through that any more.' And she came home with her driver's licence! I was crying, everybody was crying — the family, the friends. Everybody cried!

Of course it didn't stop there.

The next problem was, my husband said, 'All her friends have got cars. She wants a car, why can't we give her a car?'

Benita didn't get the sports car she wanted but a small four-door sedan, her parents having in mind that when she drove, she would always have at least one, if not two, supervising passengers with her. But that didn't last forever. It was a while before Ana ceased to feel anxious (even taking to following Benita when she went out in the car by herself) but in time she recognised Benita's capacity to cope: 'She amazes me every day.'

On the other hand, there's often a friend with a car, which can have its advantages, as Alex Major discovered.

Jan: Tell me, when you go out to the Metropolis [night club] in Fremantle, how do you get there and how do you get home?
Alex: Andrew gives us a lift.
Jan: He drives?
Alex: He drives, so he can't drink too much. He drinks water and soft drink mainly.
Jan: Do you like to drink?
Alex: I drink, like, beer, wine, whisky, bourbon. Anything that's really a high alcohol level!

If young people with Down syndrome don't learn to drive — and certainly the majority don't at present — then transport usually devolves onto the parents. Transport training, making people independent in terms of public transport, is a big issue. Many high schools with education support facilities offer transport training as part of the package of survival skills they try to introduce to their students; other people learn this through work experience or employment support agencies. Others are simply thrown in.

Lucy Burton goes to high school not far from home in Perth's western suburbs, and from the time she started secondary school has been catching the regular bus. Her mother Heather took it for granted.

> I just made her do it. I gave her one lesson. I just went down there and took the bus home. And of course there are other kids from the school on that same bus, even though there are other members of the public, but she crosses the highway by herself, and I just hope for the best, because apparently she has been seen dancing on the median strip with her iPod, and people were worried that she was going to get killed. But anyway that seems to have ironed itself out, because I told her she's not to do that. That's one thing about Lucy, if I really ram it home to her that she is *not* to do something and why, she usually complies, so that's good ...

> But you realise there are things about buses that you just take for granted, things that you actually have to learn, like one day — because Lucy thinks, 'I live in Perth' — she got on the bus, thinking she was being very clever, and asks, 'Oh, do you go to Perth?' The driver said, 'No, you'd better get off.' So she got off and it was actually the right bus, because there's only one bus anyway from that stop. So then she's up in the office at school crying, saying, 'Oh, wrong bus,' and

then I get the phone call, and I said, 'Well, just put her on the next bus.' Then another time she missed the bus from home to school, so then she comes home crying, not realising that there is another one in ten minutes. So things like that — you've got to learn that they do keep coming.

Sometimes parents found that their efforts to teach their children to exercise responsibility were frustrated by other people who did not understand the implications of their well-intentioned intervention. Penny Innes recalled an incident when her daughter Rebecca was undertaking her traineeship at a local council.

She missed the bus one day and the supervisor drove her home. They should have actually phoned the support worker, or helped her get the next bus, but they didn't. So, of course, Rebecca thought this was wonderful, missed the bus quite a few times after that until I actually said to the supervisor, 'Well I'm really sorry, but no.' So next time she missed the bus she went into a friend's shop and I had a call from the friend saying, 'Rebecca's here, shall I bring her home?' I said, 'No. Nobody will give her a lift. Just make sure she walks up to her bus stop.' 'Shall I give her something to eat or drink?' I said, 'No, just sit her outside and tell her when she has to go.' The next minute Rebecca had disappeared, and somebody else, another friend rang me and said, 'I've got Rebecca with me, shall I drive her home?' About three people had seen her, it was just one of those days that people saw her. I said, 'No, the best thing you can do is make sure she gets on that bus and then I'll be happy.' She got home and said, 'I'm really tired, Mum.' I said, 'Well, don't miss the bus again, will you?' and she hasn't. I was really horrible. But she hasn't done it again. That's the only way you can do it, you've got to be really firm, and that's what they should do at work.

Penny and Rebecca lived in a small town outside Perth where they were both well known. For most parents though, tough love can be a little harder on Perth's busy streets, and some parents found their children's behaviour simply too challenging even to contemplate encouraging the independence Penny Innes and Heather Burton successfully fostered in their daughters. Bernard Grant's son Angus is in his thirties and has had the benefit of some limited public transport training but his work placements since leaving school were not conducive to using public transport, and his limited verbal skills added to his parents' concern for his wellbeing and inhibited the development of independence.

There was a period when at Bentley we did get some help, because I think he was more or less on the bus run for one of their Activ workshops, so he got on that bus. But that dried up eventually and we had to get back into doing it ourselves. Angela is even concerned about him going in taxis, so even though we've got the taxi voucher scheme, we've hardly ever used that. So I think in some ways he could have been a bit more independent. We've been a bit too fearful of letting him. I think Angela's concerns are justified to some extent, because he's a bit dangerous by himself. When I'm crossing the street with traffic, he'll just sort of look straight across. I push his head, and say, 'Look that way. It's dangerous what you're doing.' Even in a parking lot he sometimes would break free and race toward the car, and he wouldn't look. So he would need more training really to be more independent in that area. (Bernard Grant)

Until the family got some assistance through an intensive family support package, the consequence was a return car run from the Perth hills where the family lived down to Angus's workplace, morning and evening, a daily total of over one hundred kilometres and a great deal of time.

Transport training typically revolves around a structured journey to a particular place such as work or school and does not necessarily lend itself to planning or undertaking an independent journey to a place of choice. Though Theresa Mansour was independent getting to and from school, then work, her mother worried about her when she made plans to meet her boyfriend.

> She has been transport trained. She was trained to take the bus to school. That was fine but I feel that I wouldn't trust her to go say up north to Perth city, because you catch another bus. It's really restricting for her and for us. Like with her boyfriend, she wants to go and visit him, she has to go to Garden City, get a bus from here to Garden City, from Garden City catch another bus to go there; then her boyfriend, he has to too. I don't trust her to go on another bus just like that.

Michael Klein travels across Perth and the suburbs to attend TAFE and work, as do Alex Major and Amelia Bakker. All three of these young people seem to be reasonably self-reliant in terms of travel. Amelia also frequently and independently makes use of the taxi voucher system to take a taxi to work or a daytime sporting or recreational activity in an otherwise inaccessible location if a family member cannot take her. However, gender undoubtedly adds a complication for parents. Rachel Kingston travels independently to work, changing from train to bus in Perth city, but her parents are not so comfortable with the thought of her taking the train to Fremantle in the evening to attend a dance class, or going out at night with a friend. As a result, her social and recreational activities tend to be confined to daylight hours and places close to home such as the gym, going to the football or shopping.

Unfortunately, things can go wrong. While still at school and actually in the company of a teacher, Laura Middleton experienced some problems on a train journey and though her words don't fully convey her emotion, she was clearly upset when she told the story. What would be a small incident of minor importance for most sixteen year olds played on her mind as a very significant event.

> **Laura**: Well it was a bit awful when I first got off the train and Nigel was in the wheelchair and Mr Cooper was trying to get the wheelchair off the train, but the doors slammed into him and it drove off.
>
> **Jan**: So what happened?
>
> **Laura**: I was actually off the train, but by myself because Mr Cooper was trying to get the wheelchair off the train, but he couldn't because the doors closed and it drove off.
>
> **Jan**: What did you do?
>
> **Laura**: Well I was waiting outside patiently and the security came and told me that they'll be back, and just to wait patiently, and I did.
>
> **Jan**: Oh that was good. But how did you feel?
>
> **Laura**: Well a bit lonely, upset and lonely.

Nicola Webb used to travel to her job at Centrelink in Gosnells on the train until she was attacked by some kids who punched her and tried to take her bag. Her father was outraged, not so much by the attack as by the indifference of the other passengers.

The kids, they just did what horrible little kids do sometimes. They were eleven year olds. The biggest problem was, the people on the train never stopped it — they just sat and watched. I mean, what threat is an eleven year old kid to any adult on the train? And they sat and watched Nic move from one chair to another, *five times*, and still let this thing go on. It was on the video on the train! Yet they want to blame the kids that were giving her a hard time! It took Steph years to get her to go on the train on her own. People don't understand how long you take to teach your kid to ride a bike, let alone get the kid to go on her own on the train. Nicola's twenty-five now and still won't go back on the train on her own. I mean I was pretty lousy about it and still am. (Paul Webb)

The incident affected not just Nicola but the whole household.

I had to give up what I was doing because she wouldn't get back on the train again. I was working for Silver Chain, so I had to give that up so I could take her to work. I just thought, well, it's more important that we do whatever we can for her, rather than do something for myself. (Steph Webb)

Three years later when Nicola started working in a different location, her family decided to renew transport training with a view to her regaining her independence. But her vulnerability remained a problem. As her father said, she was just 'Fair game, poor little Nicola, because she's not as tall as some of the kids, maybe they think she's younger than she is.'

Every family and every individual makes decisions — sometimes hard ones — about balancing the dignity of risk against an understanding of individual vulnerability and capacity to deal with things that go wrong. These choices are also weighed against how the individual's needs fit in with the needs of the family, as was the case for Nicola's family. Other mothers, like Trish Weston, similarly commented on the impact of their children's timetable.

> Will arrives home from work at 2.30 p.m. so we have to ensure someone is home at that time for him. I'm not sure how we would manage if we worked nine to five.

Theresa Mansour's family was grateful for her work and her full calendar of recreational activities, including church, social club outings, pilates, swimming, and tennis in summer, but if transport wasn't included in these activities, then her family had to take her.

> It gets a bit exhausting because you can't plan your day. If she goes out we have to be here when she goes and we have to be here when she comes back, and with her work because it's every day at 11.30, it also tends to cut into your day. You know it's hard to plan a holiday, but we cope. (Claudia Mansour)

Parents with no family backup simply have to make alternative arrangements work, which can impact particularly heavily on single parents. Grace Harvey has had her own door key since she was fifteen and is sometimes dropped off after school to wait for her mother Brenda to come home. Michael Klein has been accustomed to spending time at home alone since he was in his mid teens and is very comfortable preparing for his own departure for work after his mother leaves home each morning. However, an individual's particular support needs and capacity for independence is a big issue.

As parents age too, they come to depend more on support services to fill gaps where they can't. The Mann family used Activ Foundation's recreation department when Geoffrey was younger and through this he participated in a huge range of activities well outside his everyday experience, including canoeing, bushwalking, windsurfing, camping, even abseiling.

> Things that we would never have thought of launching Geoffrey into and he loves it. The challenge is terrific! It's really excellent for him, because it offers him a variety of recreational activities. But we're very dependent now on the recreation department to give Geoffrey the physical activity that he needs because we're getting too old to run round pushing him on a bike! (William Mann)

Geoffrey also participated in a number of national and international tours with Activ, as did Christine Conway and Geraldine Howe, two young women who lived together in their shared unit. But these things all cost money, as Claudia Mansour pointed out, and can become quite a financial burden on the family or the individual.

> Theresa gets the pension, it's a bit reduced because she is earning some money at the hospital, in her work, but I mean you calculate all of this, it doesn't leave too much.

Social life for young adults with Down syndrome also takes on a new complexion once they leave school. And again, gender makes a difference, with parents predictably more protective of their daughters, though also aware of their sons' vulnerability. Family, particularly siblings of the same gender, can play a significant role in the social lives of people with Down syndrome, with clothes shopping, movies, clubbing, pub nights, sports events and concerts all activities where sibling support features heavily. Catherine Franklin's elder sister Louisa organised Catherine's twenty-first birthday party, which was, according to mother Pamela, 'the best party of all time I tell you,' and Catherine is the weekly 'cheer squad and coach' for Louisa's basketball games. The sisters frequently shop together and Louisa and her friends often include Catherine in their activities.

> Though Catherine can be a little bit of a shit from time to time. Louisa takes her to the pub and her friends are all fantastic and they all look after her, but Catherine will dump Louisa if someone else is more interesting. She doesn't have the sensibility to know that if it wasn't for Louisa, her life would be seriously curtailed, but Louisa's big enough to handle all that. (Pamela Franklin)

Laura Middleton's elder sister Ruth has also been a mainstay of Laura's 'special events' social life, having taken her to see a number of big shows including Christina Aguilera and 'a fantastic concert by Justin Timberlake, the Future Sex Love Show' at Burswood Dome. James Austen's elder brothers took him out for his first beer when he turned eighteen.

Friendship and social life remain a concern for parents as their kids grow up. A number of parents commented that open employment workplaces had not become a source of friendships outside work and in fact, could be quite lonely environments. For that reason, some parents who might have preferred to see their children face the challenges of open employment opted for disability enterprises instead. The situation paralleled that of inclusive versus 'special' or segregated education and Virginia Robb, who was turned off educational inclusion by her daughter's experience of tokenistic mainstreaming, had thought at length about friendship and workplace inclusion.

I initially thought that the best thing would be for her to be able to work in a mainstream office or something, but there's a girl with Down syndrome at netball that Georgia plays with, a great kid, twenty-one or something — her mum said that sometimes it's lonely for her because she doesn't get invited out with the other office workers. So she's kind of betwixt and between. I had a long talk to Georgia's high school teacher about this and she said, 'You have to be very careful about it, because when they get into the workforce, it's great to have the skills to work in a mainstream job, but the reality sometimes is that those friendships don't blossom and develop because at the end of the day who's going to invite the kid with disabilities down to the pub on a Friday night, whereas if she goes into something like Activ or where there's other people with disabilities, you'd be surprised, they have a great time. They're social, they go out together.' So what we think is best for the kids isn't necessarily what the kids need. That was a hard thing for me, I think, to accept that, because you want your child to be as normal as possible, but at the end of the day they're not.

Many of Theresa Mansour's colleagues from the hospital where she works came to her twenty-first birthday party, but on the whole, friendships seem to develop more naturally among people who work in disability enterprises. Social activities though seem less likely to revolve around work than around hobbies and old school friends. While some adults with Down syndrome such as Charlie King, Frank Flynn and Sandra Rossi, all in the Kimberley, have little or no contact with other people with Down syndrome, in metropolitan areas young adults tend to socialise fairly frequently with others with Down syndrome or other disabilities. Catherine

Franklin has two particular friends with whom she went to school, both of whom have Down syndrome. All are in their early twenties and they regularly socialise together, though their freedom is still carefully monitored by their parents.

> Most weekends the three of them will be together and they'll go down to Claremont and they'll have a drink, and they'll have coffee and they'll go and look at all the shops. Walk down, walk back, and more often than not they'll stay here on Saturday night if nothing else is happening. They'll have a video night or they listen to music. They do like going out though, they love going out. We took the three of them down to Fremantle the other Saturday and they just loved that, for dinner, and then we went to Time Zone. They love that sort of thing.

> They wouldn't go down to Fremantle on a Saturday night by themselves though, just the three of them, because it's too dangerous. Because if some smarmy bloke came along they'd think that's pretty good, that sort of thing. So they are vulnerable, and no, I wouldn't let them go. Catherine would like to think that some bloke thought she was great or something and I can imagine her falling for what he might say. So that is a problem. (Pamela Franklin)

Helen Golding made the same point regarding her youngest daughter.

> Josie is going to be easily taken advantage of because she really likes people; she still is over-friendly despite the fact that she has been taught for years that she needs not to be, which is another reason why she is going to need supervision for the rest of her life because she will put herself at risk.

Friendships and social networks for young people with Down syndrome in their mid to late teens usually focused on old school friends and recreational contacts, though as Luke Middleton acknowledged, his daughter Laura's friendships were increasingly with other people with disabilities, and his partner Jude agreed with his reservations about this.

> **Luke:** She's got a big bunch of friends, all kids with disabilities. I would love Laura to have friends outside of those kids, but they're the kids she feels comfortable with, and they feel comfortable with her and they're all close friends.
>
> **Jude:** Yes, I love Laura's friends, but I think the whole world out there is not disabled. It would be good for her to socialise with other people and it would be good for other kids too if they'd become accustomed to kids with disabilities, but that's not happening, it's really not.

Ana Diaz's concern was that her daughter Benita had few friends of her own age at all, with or without disabilities.

> She really enjoys friends, Benita enjoys friends, but normal people as friends. But she's always with old people, she's always with us. I mean, we go to our club, they have dancing once a month, but old people. The young people don't go anymore. And I wish that I could say, okay, I'd like to go to the club, and she could go somewhere else. She can have her friends, she can have somewhere to go. I can't find any. All my life, I have been looking for a friend for her. Never find them. They are lonely people. They are.

Alison Austen's friendship strategy was to ensure her son maintained contact with a network of people with Down syndrome, in his school years and beyond.

Because even though we pursued — and you do have to work at it — friendships with the other regular kids, it's not the same. You do realise at some point that there's an affinity with other kids who have the same or similar disability in that they can relate in a totally different way. James was most happy I suppose when he was able to relax with someone else, one of his mates.

For that reason, quite a few young adults, such as Angus Grant, Nicola Webb, Christine Conway, Geraldine Howe and Amelia Bakker, participated in recreation groups organised specifically for people with disabilities.

Many young adults with Down syndrome are very much involved in non-disabled sport and recreational activities, though once again, it is generally the parents who facilitate this in the first instance. James Austen trains and swims competitively; Laura Middleton does ballroom dancing and Benita Diaz Spanish dancing; Rebecca Innes does yoga and belly dancing; Alex Major tae kwon do and Mark Brookton motocross. Nicola Webb goes with her mother to an Aboriginal women's cultural group in a suburb close to their Perth home. Others are passionate sports fans and club members. While these activities do not always spontaneously generate friendships, they do, as Ana's comments suggest, introduce people with Down syndrome to a wider range of regular opportunities and increasingly heighten both the visibility of people with disabilities and community recognition of their interests and capacities. This can break down social inhibitions and awkwardness in both directions. Will Weston, a young man with limited speech, has been riding observed trials at a motor bike club for years.

He's very much accepted in the club. The thing that people found quite hard though, to start with, is that Will wasn't speaking back to them when they said hello. So Michael said to them, 'Look, you know, he's very shy and he also finds it hard to speak, so don't stop saying hello to him. Keep including him and keep saying hello and eventually it will work out fine.' Now Will does either gesture or say hello back to people, and has basic sorts of conversations when they ask him things. People have kept on trying to do that. He fits in really well and people are always glad to see him, so it's great. Oh yes, he's very much accepted. (Trish Weston)

Perhaps, as the following chapter discusses, deeper community engagement might eventually follow.

Another critical moment for young people with Down syndrome is puberty, though sometimes parents — perhaps unconsciously — suppress the associated thought of their child becoming a sexualised being and an adult. This attitude partly stems from an understanding of people with Down syndrome as leading a life of perpetual childhood, long evident in the literature about people with intellectual disabilities, from Pearl Buck's *The Child Who Never Grew*, to Brazilian Cristovão Tezza's recently translated book about Down syndrome, *The Eternal Son*. A girl, especially one with an intellectual disability, may be a woman in a physical sense when she starts to menstruate but emotionally and developmentally she often still seems a child. Jude Lawrence recalled the circumstances when her eldest daughter Ruth realised with a shock that her younger sister with Down syndrome was going to grow up.

Ruth and I went to the Down Syndrome Congress in Singapore in 2004, and it was really good for Ruth because there were lots of young adults with Down syndrome wandering around and she met and talked to quite a few young people with Down syndrome. But she also saw people from all over the world getting together and, you know, walking around holding hands. She was amazed and she said, 'I've just never thought about people with Down syndrome having relationships.' And we met some people there whose adult children with Down syndrome were married, so that was a bit of a revelation for her too. She's now seeing that Laura is a person who will grow up to have a relationship, we hope, and maybe live with someone who she will possibly marry, who will love her, and be loved by her. It was a real reminder to us all that you're not dealing with someone who will always be a child.

While people with Down syndrome are exposed as much as most people to sexuality, especially through the media, their understanding of emotions and relationships is likely to be even more limited than it is for other teenagers. Knowing how to deal directly with the subject of sex and their children's sexuality was often difficult for parents, so courses on sexuality run by organisations such as People First and SECCA (Sexuality Education Counselling & Consultancy Agency), which many teenagers access through school and which focus on appropriate and protective behaviours, were a great boon to parents. William Mann for instance had not discussed sex with Geoffrey.

There was a course, one of the first TAFE courses for people with disabilities and I think he did it twice, and there was some social trainer who talked about the idea of a 'circle of friends', that you attached different degrees of affection to people within different circles, and I think he understood that. And this is one of the problems we had, with respect to him going up to girls and hugging them and stroking their hair. And we had to explain to him that you didn't do that sort of thing to strangers. You can do it to your sisters, and with good friends you shake hands. But that's the extent of my involvement in that sort of discussion.

With her three adolescent children, Helen Golding had a lot of emergent sexuality to cope with all at once.

The two older ones are very sexually aware, Damian probably more than Charlotte, and through school, he did the People First program, which is very good from a point of view of covering the tintacks of 'This is a condom and this is what you do with it,' but I have some concerns about the level of values and stress on relationships that is a part of that program. I have always stressed with the kids that you have sex with someone who you are married to preferably. But I don't put in the 'preferably' when I am talking to them. So that they have some understanding that it is not just something that you go out and do, you know. 'I am old enough now, I will go and do it, I am eighteen, I can go and have a beer, I am eighteen, I can go and have sex with the fellows.' So that they have some understanding that there is more to this than what you see on TV. Charlotte certainly seems to understand that that is the way it is. Damian talks big but I think he also understands that sexuality is something that is private and that it is part of a relationship and it is not something that you just go out and do because you feel like it. Being sixteen he likes to talk about it and watching TV, he likes to say, '*I think they are going to have sex,*' just because he likes the excuse to use the words I think.

People with Down syndrome are generally as keen on growing up sexually and, given the opportunity, as apt to fall in love as anyone else, like James Austen.

He's always been interested in having a girlfriend, that just seems to be par for the course. He was at high school and suddenly he was surrounded by girls and a new world opened up — wow, you know, I can be a boy, I can kiss a girl and I can hold her hand, and I can put my arm around her! Actually, depending on who he was with at the time, he'd get up close and personal any chance he'd get! So he tried all those things like most boys do, only he was more obvious than everybody else and while they did it on the quiet he did it in full view! I think it was good training for him really ...

Before he found his first steady girlfriend shortly after leaving high school, James experienced a lot of crushes and at least one broken heart.

He was just desperately, madly in love with Alicia and asked her to the ball and that was his first date and he thought that that meant they were together forever. There were a lot of lessons learned about what makes two people boyfriend and girlfriend. (Alison Austen)

His parents recognised the need for him to meet a broader group of friends, male and female, because as his mother said, 'his horizons are so limited in lots of ways.' Consequently James joined a social group for young people with Down syndrome where he met his girlfriend Verity.

For the eighteen months he was going to the social group he used to see Verity every Saturday and that was lovely because it was something that grew. And then the group finished and it was two or three weeks and he hadn't actually asked to see her, but I don't think he realised he could. He was just getting sadder and wanted to see her. We helped him express that, and Verity's mother and I talked and we were able to make it easy for them to see each other. So we facilitated that. Now you can see the sun shining out of him because he's found a girl who adores him and he adores her, and they can't wait till they see each other next time, and they write each other emails and it's just lovely. (Alison Austen)

James was nineteen, his girlfriend a little older. If things were different they would have been spending a lot of time together, driving to places, going out at night clubbing or for a drink. For young people with disabilities however there is often a need for parents to play an overt role in nurturing a relationship, setting up contacts and social networks in the first place, arranging transport, especially in a city as tied to the use of private cars as Perth is, and perhaps supervising activities, recognising issues and dealing with them. And again, if things were different, this young couple might also have begun thinking of the future, despite their youth, but this seemed a long way outside James's world view. He did not see himself getting married until he was fifty-four, though he thought he would like to move in with his girlfriend's family before then. He was also fairly clear that longer term he would prefer to keep living with a family, rather than alone with Verity.

Michael Klein, a young man in his mid twenties, has been going out with nineteen year old Jessica, who also has Down syndrome, since they met at TAFE a couple of years ago. He has had a couple of girlfriends before, though as he says, it is 'hard to get girls,' but she is his first serious girlfriend and Michael has a true romantic's understanding of the important things in a relationship.

Stuff like looking at the stars, looking at the sunset, walking on the beach, having dinner, a nice picnic lunch. Valentine's

Day this year I had dinner with her in Fremantle and we went to see the movie *Valentine's Day* and I bought red roses and a card for her.

Michael considers Jessica as 'one of the young ones' and is very conscious of the need to protect her, escorting her home on the bus from Fremantle where they often meet. They frequently see each other in the company of Jessica's family or Michael's parents. Michael is also helping Jessica to learn skills such as money handling and independent transport. Though he has many of these skills himself he and Jessica both recently enrolled in an Activ course on independent living, particularly for Jessica's benefit. As for the future, though his boss says, 'When are we going to see you in Church?' and some of his friends on Facebook are also asking him when they are getting married, Michael's philosophy is, 'Take it easy, take your time, no rush, it's new for me and new for her.' He is keeping up with his old friends and contacts, though he and Jessica see each other most days, and as he says, the relationship has made him 'very very happy.'

As relationships progress, the issue of contraception may also arise, a particularly fraught area for parents of daughters with intellectual disabilities. A number of the young women in this book were already using the contraceptive pill, but for managing heavy periods rather than for contraception. Doctors had also raised with some mothers the use of Depo Provera and the Mirena IUD for menstrual management but other than heavy bleeding, few of the young women had any particular problems coping with the normal routine of menstruation. A number of parents had viewed very explicit films on menstruation with their daughters, which they found excellent. Some education support classes in schools also introduced high school girls early on to the idea of managing menstruation by, for example, having them wear sanitary pads on excursions and teaching them how to dispose of them at school and in public facilities.

In terms of the need for contraception however, though a number of the people with Down syndrome I spoke to had had a boyfriend or girlfriend, none suggested they were or had been in a sexual relationship, one of the older women telling me very bluntly that she was a virgin when I asked her if she had had a 'serious' boyfriend. Thus the question of contraception did not generally come up in my conversations with the women themselves. But the big issue for most parents was, if their daughter had a baby, who would look after it? Though almost every parent expressed their belief that they would love to see their child with a life partner, married or otherwise, only one advocated the right of her daughter to have a child if she wanted. Some young women told me directly they would like to have children (Eloise Hartley wanted four); but a number of mothers had adopted a conscious policy of pointing out friends with no children and setting them up as role models, or actively reminding their daughters at every opportunity, including during our interview, as Steph Webb did, just how much hard work children are to look after.

> **Steph**: Nicola doesn't want to have kids, do you Nic?
> **Nicola**: No.
> **Steph**: Too much hard work to look after. Because you wouldn't like to look after Ruby all the time would you? Would you like to look after her all the time?
> **Nicola**: No.
> **Steph**: No. It's too much hard work, isn't it Nic?

A couple of the mothers I spoke to felt quite strongly that sterilisation would be an appropriate means of avoiding pregnancy in their daughter's case. Sterilisation has deep and unpleasant associations in the history of disability, and sterilisation without consent for non-therapeutic reasons is illegal in Australia, although recent reports confirm that it happens in reasonably high numbers.[110] One woman put the pro-sterilisation case from a mother's point of view.

> I don't honestly think she'd be able to cope, having a child, or looking after a child ... Oh I'd be all for sterilisation, for sure. I've spoken to our doctor and they're not too keen on things like that, because they say kids with disabilities have got a right to say yes or no. But then I think as parents we really should have that right over them because we're the one that's got to deal with it. I mean I don't want to be left looking after a grandchild, because I've had my life and I just honestly wouldn't be able to cope doing that. I think as parents we should be allowed to make that decision. It's okay for them up there to say, 'Oh they should do this and that,' but they don't live with a child with a disability 24/7, so they really don't know what it's like. It's all right for the bureaucrats to say, 'Oh they've got rights,' yes, they do have rights with certain things, but then I think parents have got rights with bringing up a child with a disability. We wouldn't be doing it because we don't want her to have a child; it's just that she wouldn't be able to cope with a child. That's just the way it is.[111]

Janet Rossi had a different perspective on the issue of rights in the case of her daughter Sandra.

> **Janet**: She's always dreamed about having a baby of her own.
> **Jan**: Have you talked to her about that as a possibility?
> **Janet**: Yes, and she knows about the birds and the bees and

stuff like that, so she's aware of it. But she became really obsessed with having a baby at one stage, and we had to keep making her face the hard reality of it, and what it's all about and that seemed to settle her down a little bit.

Jan: How would you feel if she met someone?

Janet: She's had her interests and things like that, in boys, like any normal girl, and she talks about it. I don't think I'd have a big issue with it. I mean I'd like her to have a normal life like anybody else when it comes to that sort of thing, but it's just a matter of finding someone that's compatible I suppose.

Jan: You wouldn't think of sterilisation?

Janet: No. Well it has crossed my mind, but I don't think I have the right to do that, although I'd probably be faced with all the headaches and the responsibilities if something did happen. Yes, it's a hard one. I mean I have looked into it before, because she was having lots of problems with her periods, really heavy bleeding. But I don't believe in giving her Depo Provera and stuff like that. I've just seen a lot of women use that and they're treated as guinea pigs and develop cancer and all sorts of things, so I wouldn't put that on her anyway. So yes, she just takes the pill.

The process of young people with Down syndrome growing up, leaving school, and generally aspiring to a more adult lifestyle, can be confronting for everyone involved. The transition to work, for instance, is not always easy but it can be made simpler for both individuals and families by careful planning ahead of time. As is the case with any child leaving school, learning what the available options are and how they fit in with a young adult's individual needs and their own perceptions of what is appropriate, is critical, though parents need to be a little more interventionist as things progress than they do with their other children. At the same time, family dynamics may need to be reassessed and the long-term significance of this new stage in a person's life considered and managed. There may still be no apparent end date on the support required for adult children with Down syndrome living at home, but the nature of that support certainly changes once school days are over. Fortunately for people with disabilities and their parents, now there are opportunities available to facilitate their leading a full and meaningful life of great activity and challenge.

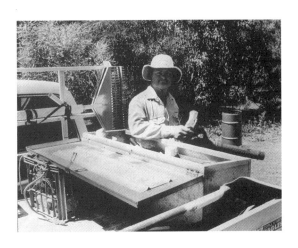

chapter 7

'WE'VE GOT TO OUTLIVE HIM!'

'The term "independent living" as defined by people with disabilities does not mean doing things for yourself, or living on your own. It means having choice and control over the assistance needed for daily life and having access to amenities that society has to offer such as housing, transport, health services, employment, as well as entertainment, education and training opportunities.'[112]

By the second half of the twentieth century, the first generation of parents who had fought to keep their children out of institutions was starting to face the longer term implications of their struggle. At a meeting called by the Slow Learning Children's Group in Perth in 1951 to discuss future accommodation options for their children, the father of a young woman with Down syndrome posed the question which still vexes parents of children with disabilities today.

What was to become of them when their parents were taken? It was and is not fair to expect other members of the family to accept this responsibility.[113]

The need for a solution to that quandary has become even more pressing in the twenty-first century. While the end of institutionalisation, and changes in health access and social attitudes, have meant that people with Down syndrome are now generally experiencing better health and enhanced life expectancy, this has not always been matched by improvements in the availability of accommodation or other support. As Trish Weston, mother of a young man in his twenties said, 'It is the sort of stage of life where you're realising that you do have to be doing some real future planning for your child.' And 'We've got to outlive him' became the mantra, only half joking, of the Manns, whose son with Down syndrome was born in the 1970s.

Faced with a child who — at least at first — they fear will never be independent, never able to manage her own affairs, never capable of protecting himself or living independently, some parents start planning the day the child is born for a future which they suspect will be bleak. For many, these fears take a back seat as the child ages, but others hold onto them to the point of irrationality and despair. In Western Australia, there have been at least two cases of young people with disabilities being killed by fathers (Joseph O'Sullivan in 1936, and the much-publicised Benn case in 1964) who were so fearful about their child's future that they deprived them of the chance to experience it.[114] In 2003, while apparently experiencing post-natal depression related in part to her child's condition, American university professor Mine Ener killed her five month old daughter with Down syndrome and subsequently committed suicide.[115] Seeing a child with a disability age without a plan in place for their safe future care, can too easily lead parents to desperation.

At the time of the Benn case, according to historian Christina Gillgren, the availability of state residential care for people with intellectual disabilities could, 'only be described as deplorable.'[116] Subsequently the provision of accommodation in Western Australia began to improve under the auspices of Guy Hamilton, whose intervention in the care of people with intellectual disabilities has meant that in many respects Western Australia has been a pioneer in the early provision of some services, including accommodation.[117] Today there are at least some options — not always perfect, not as accessible as parents might like, but there is certainly more reason to hope that people with Down syndrome born in the last few decades will be able to live a decent well-rounded life as they age, without the constant need for intervention and monitoring by parents and siblings. This chapter explores some of the options which have emerged over the past two decades, and looks at how people with disabilities and their family members have worked towards achieving adult independence.

For parents of a child with a disability, planning for the future means planning for a place where their child can live independently. But what exactly does 'independent living' mean in this context? Some of the people interviewed in this book, like Jeremy Young and Rebecca Innes, live in their own homes, by themselves or with a partner or friend, with minimal intervention from outsiders; others require more support.

For Bernard Grant, 'independent living' for his son Angus meant living apart from his parents, in the community, in a situation with continuity where he was secure, respected and safe; an understanding underpinned by recognition of the need for continuing support.

I think Angus'll always need 24/7 care of one sort or another, but I would hope for him that he could continue to do the things he really enjoys and continue to have a good strong social life, with people who value him.

Bernard's idea of 'independence' transcended simply having a place to live, and encompassed 'having a fulfilled life and good friends around him, finding work that's meaningful and useful, and good recreational opportunities.'

Trish Weston similarly understood independence for her son in broad terms of living safely, securely and happily, and with people he could relate to.

We really hope he will have a place in society that he will be respected. I don't have a problem with him living with perhaps a group of other people with intellectual disabilities at all. I know that some people say, 'Oh no, that's really not the way that other people live.' But it is; you gravitate towards those people that you relate to the best, and I would certainly like him to have friends that are not intellectually disabled, but at the same time I want him to be with those people that he feels most comfortable with. I want him to be happy more than anything else and if that's what he wants, then that's what we want. And, of course, I want his safety too. So I would have to make sure that wherever he is there is the amount of supervision that he will require to be safe.

So 'independent living' is far more complex than simply living apart from one's family or without any assistance or intervention. It is about living within a larger community environment which is sustaining, even nurturing; being respected for one's abilities and gifts; and undertaking activities, paid and unpaid, which give life meaning. As the Disability Services Commission website says, it's about 'a good life.'[118]

Leading a good life typically entails some concerted planning on the part of the parents, starting with an acknowledgement that having a child move out of the family home is ultimately beneficial for both the parents and the individual. The decision can be approached gradually, or it can be forced upon a family by circumstances beyond its control. It can be couched in terms of what is best for the child, for the parents, or for the larger family. It can be painful, it's seldom undertaken lightly, and it can be postponed almost indefinitely. But even those parents who laugh and say, 'Oh, she'll be living with us forever,' eventually have to confront the reality of their own mortality.

Sometimes a change in family circumstances or a new job opportunity can accelerate the process of a son or daughter moving out. The Mann family had always envisaged that their son would leave home, but this occurred rather sooner than the family anticipated.

In the early 1980s, when Geoffrey was about twenty-five, I had a bout of illness and I was rather disgusted to find that, although everybody in AIH [Authority for Intellectually Handicapped Persons] and Activ knew of my illness because they sent cards and flowers and fruit and so forth, nobody did anything for Geoffrey. When I came out of hospital I rang up Irrabeena and virtually said, 'Well where's this much flaunted crisis care you're talking about?' 'Oh dear, dear! What do you want us to do?' 'Well, it isn't a matter of what I want to do,' I said, 'It's a matter of what Geoffrey wants, and he wants to live in a group home.' 'Oh well, now that's a problem because of the shortage of places.' However, some six or eight weeks later, they found a place in a group home for Geoffrey and he was enchanted to go. (Muriel Mann)

When Richie Stevens was in his forties, his parents' health issues necessitated the break-up of the household he had lived in north of Perth all his life. His mother had developed Parkinson's and his father Alzheimer's, and both required permanent care, leaving Richie's sister Jill Mather, four hundred kilometres south, largely responsible for all three. The most stable arrangement for Richie was to continue living in the family home, a beach house which had once been a temporary summer home for the family but which had become the family's permanent residence when Richie was in his twenties. Working through a local community living group, Jill found Richie a full-time live-in carer who was funded through grants available through the government disability service network. Richie also has an outside mentor who visits him once or twice a week and arranges social activities such as bowling. The situation is stable, though expensive in terms of support, and when I talked to them all, Jill, Richie and Richie's carer Gordon Griffith were investigating the prospect of Richie sharing a home — his or someone else's — with another person with a disability.

In some cases, young people with Down syndrome are themselves the instigators of the move out of the family home. By the time she was sixteen, Eloise Hartley had left her Catholic girls school where she had been part of a reasonably inclusive program, and was attending a city TAFE and undertaking pre-apprenticeship training in child care and hairdressing. She travelled independently to TAFE, as she had done to school, using public transport and changing from buses to trains, and even before her parents were ready, had begun planning for an independent future away from home. Her two older sisters had already left home and she had a younger brother with whom, she said, she fought 'constantly'. She was ready to go. Perhaps her plans, as she outlined them at the age of sixteen, sounded a little naive: 'Well, I have to leave home one day. I might live in an apartment in a hotel or something.' But when I interviewed her again just a few years later, Eloise's vision had materialised. She and her friend Rachel, who also has Down syndrome, were living in a two-bedroom unit owned by Eloise's parents in a central Perth location. While their parents provided some support, the young women were largely independent.

An individual leaving home has to be ready both physically and emotionally for the move, and so do parents. Difficult as it may sometimes be to push any young adult out the door, some parents find this immeasurably harder to do if their daughter or son has a disability — not because the child doesn't want to go but because the parents don't want them to. This was very clear in my conversation with Ana Diaz and her daughter Benita, who was in her late twenties.

> **Jan** (to Ana): Have you ever thought about Benita moving out from the family home here?
>
> **Ana**: We're all right at the moment, we handle it all right, I don't think she will be going. But she says, you know, 'I want to go.'
>
> **Benita**: I want to be free. I want to be free.
>
> **Ana**: See, she knows how to do a lot of things. Yes. I think she could. I don't worry about her ... The only thing that worries me is ... when I go, what would happen. That worries me, yes.
>
> **Benita**: No problem at all.
>
> **Ana**: No problem at all, she thinks she is going to be all right.
>
> **Benita**: I told you I would and that's it. Oh, come on Mum!
>
> **Ana**: She's very good company. I mean when she is home, and the music on, and dancing ...

Benita: I enjoy myself.

Ana: But when we are by ourselves, it's like an empty house.

Benita: It's not an empty house!

Ana: Like an empty house.

The conflict between head and heart was similarly apparent for Paul Webb.

We'd love to have her with us always but some day Nicola may well be better off somewhere else, doing her own little thing instead of say, making Dad a cup of coffee or cleaning up the dishes, or doing this or that. But it's hard to accept that one day she will be living somewhere else.

On the other hand, like Michael Klein, young people themselves may have their own reasons for wanting to stay at home.

Jan: Do you ever think you might like to live by yourself, or with a friend or something like that?

Michael: I don't know. I don't think Mum will give me issues about, like if I have a girlfriend. But I prefer to be home. If Mum died, or if she had a heart attack or something, I would do something, I'd help her. I'd save her life.

Anna Klein: If I had a heart attack you would try and save me, would you?

Michael: Yes. I remember on the news when I was a kid, bathing, a swimming pool. A hero saved a friend or whatever. I am going to do that.

Michael's responsible attitude towards his mother, a single parent, was undoubtedly influenced by the fact that he had lost his elder brother in an accident and he now saw himself as her sole support. In fact 'interdependence' cuts both ways and is another aspect of having an ageing person with Down syndrome remain at home. A person with Down syndrome may be able to give sufficient support to older parents to enable them to continue living in their own home longer than would otherwise be the case.[119]

Location and gender can both influence the way individual parents feel about their child leaving home. Wendy and Keith Brookton, living in a small town in the far north of the state, had no doubts that their son would live independently. In fact they were bringing up Mark, like all their children, to be independent and self-sufficient and didn't envisage him having any choice in the matter! But they were also comfortable that their community was a supportive one where he would find employment and respect.

Jan: You place a big emphasis on independence for Mark. What do you think his prospects are for living independently in the future?
Wendy: He's going to have to; he's not living with us!
Jan: When do you think he'll move out?
Wendy: Eighteen's the deadline — we've told all our kids.
Keith: If you're not out by eighteen, boy, you're gone!
Jan: You see him staying in the Kimberley?
Keith: Don't know. The girls might take off; he might take off, who knows? But I think the future's pretty good for Mark like that. I think the community's good for him too, just people in the community.

As well as being emotionally prepared for the move out (in many cases more difficult for the parent than for the child), a young adult leaving home needs to acquire at least some basic skills, a process taken fairly seriously by most parents. With a son or daughter without a disability, a parent can afford to assume they will 'manage' or simply learn by experience, but it's harder to be complacent with a person with a disability who does not perhaps have the resources to hop in the car and duck out to the laundromat or for takeaway, or to ring up a 'flying domestic'. There is also the huge issue of preparing people with disabilities to use and manage their own finances. And above all, there is the overwhelming worry about personal safety and security. So it isn't a straightforward process, and indeed, the seeming enormity of the task, combined with the very real preference for keeping this particular child 'safe' and close, often hinders progress towards independence. I asked Pamela Franklin how she would feel about her twenty-one year old daughter Catherine continuing to live at home.

> I hope she doesn't, but not for our sake. I think we will probably miss her when she goes but obviously we are not going to be around so she really needs to be as independent as could be as soon as possible. I think probably the most *likely* outcome is some sort of supervised care. Independent living, supervised independent living. I don't know whether she will ever be responsible enough to remember whether or not the gas has been left on, or the electricity or the heating and those sorts of things. I know they can learn but ... they just keep having to remember.

In his twenties, Michael Klein participated in a program facilitated through Disability Services Commission that was designed to develop independent living skills. At the education support centre he had attended at a government high school, and through TAFE, he had already begun to develop practical skills such as cooking; now household management was the next step.

Michael: On Wednesday our dear friend Roger helps me to do the shopping and cooking. I get a recipe, I'm learning to do like meatloaf or chicken fry.

Anna Klein: The idea with Roger is they've got a program where they come and teach young people, young adults, who are more or less ready to live on their own, to learn to budget and to do some simple cooking. Simple things that can be done in one pot, or one casserole. It's about ten sessions we have. So he comes every Wednesday morning, from ten to about twelve. Each week when he comes, they decide what to do the next week. Roger has designed a shopping list with pictures, but Michael prefers actually just to write down what he needs. But this is more like a trigger thing. Like one day when he's by himself, living by himself, he'll be able to go through the pictures, and say, 'Oh yes, I need that and I need that.' Then they go shopping and he has his money, his board money that he uses, and then they do a bit of cooking and I come home and have dinner cooked, which is wonderful.

Prior to Geoffrey leaving home, the Manns had some help from Irrabeena with independence training.

I certainly should give them credit for this on independence training. And they'd been offering Geoffrey, I think it was two hours a week, and it really worked miracles, you know. They expected more of him than I had. They expected him to be able to vacuum his room and operate the washing machine, do his own ironing, handle his own pension money, allocate it to all the different things that he would require — money for swimming, money for Discovery Club, and money for dancing. (Muriel Mann)

The Goldings had three children to think about and though they recognised that each one would require individual planning — there was no 'one size fits all' solution — from the time the children were in their early teens the parents had a single aim for them ten years hence.

Part of our plan includes long-term planning for assistance with independence training. The fact is, we would like them to leave home. We envisage that the three children will be living independently without us. At that stage they would be in their twenties and we think it is reasonable that they would no longer be sharing a house with us. Because we believe it is not in their best interests or ours to have them at home forever and that in their twenties they shouldn't have to be living the lifestyle of people who are in their sixties.

Having — or being — an ageing 'child' with a disability at home can certainly impact on everybody concerned, as Trish Weston reflected rather wistfully.

We look around at our friends who don't have kids with disabilities and their lives are different, there's no question about it. If we do want to go somewhere, either just one of us goes or we've got to arrange for someone to be here. For our next holiday we're planning on going down south and doing some hiking and there will be three of us, it won't be just the two of us. We love having Will around, but it still isn't the same and he wouldn't want to be around us if he didn't have a disability.

The other side of the coin from living the lifestyle of one's ageing parents is being treated like a perpetual child, as Muriel Mann recognised.

We used to always use the Slow Learning Children's Group Sitter Service when Geoffrey was young, and other teenagers around the district. But came one year when we were using the services of a colleague's daughter who was born in the same week as Geoffrey, and we thought, now this is absolutely insulting to Geoffrey, to be bringing in someone his own age to look after him. She's a very nice lass and Geoffrey loved to have her come and play ping-pong with him. He thought it was Christmas every time she came, but after that, with short absences, we tended to leave him on his own. And we discovered he enjoyed that. He thought he was king of the castle while we weren't here! The only disaster that could happen was if someone from outside impinges upon Geoffrey. I don't know that he could handle unexpected intrusion, but himself, he's quite competent to leave alone.

Many families plan to build an extra room, add a granny flat, or buy a unit or apartment where their child will live when the time comes to officially leave home. Some, like my own family, have been working towards this for years. Financial security is another issue to consider. Pamela Franklin began to discuss her daughter's continuing financial needs with her family when Catherine was still a teenager.

We have been talking about making out a will and actually I said to David that we should leave everything to her and not the other children because they are all well able to look after themselves and he was absolutely horrified. And he said, 'Oh well you know that is discriminating,' and I said, 'Well you know we have spent heaps of money on them, given them a good education, they will all be able to go out and support themselves. Otherwise they're going to be responsible.' My son said that he agreed with that. It didn't worry him.

Alongside, even transcending the question of where a family member with a disability would actually live and how they would pay for it, the provision of daily social, personal and moral support was a major concern for parents. Physical separation from siblings and parents but with some back-up family support or oversight seemed the best longer term solution for some families. The Brooktons introduced the idea constructively from early on.

> **Keith**: I've had a few talks with his sister along the lines of 'You might be able to help Mark out with a few issues later on in life.'
> **Wendy**: Money management.
> **Keith**: Yes, not really doing the Down syndrome thing, but just saying that there'll be things that he'll struggle with, there'll be things that you struggle with, but the things that he struggles with, you might be able to help him. She feels good about that.

Claudia Mansour found her family more than willing to continue to play a major role in her daughter Theresa's life.

> My children are fully prepared to have her on board and not let her go anywhere; she will have their full support. They will be there for her. They get really upset when I say, 'I don't know what's happening in the future for Theresa.' My son and my daughter — and I have a great son-in-law too, he says to me, 'You don't have to worry about Theresa.' If she chooses to be independent, I would like her to be independent and I brought her up to be independent, but she would always have our family's support.

Despite these positive assertions from siblings, many parents were reluctant to see their other children left with this responsibility. Yet the reality was that while a person with a disability lived at home, this was often already happening. Sometimes an individual's special needs impacted on the lives of the whole family, often assuming greater prominence as the family grew up.

> We try not to let this happen, but there's no question that there are times when we have to say to our daughters, 'Can you make sure that you're home by such-and-such a time, because we won't be here and Will will be here by himself for a couple of hours by then.' Whenever anyone says, 'I want to go out and do this,' we all sort of think, okay, who's going to be here with Will? (Trish Weston)

Parents were also torn between the hope that their other children would 'naturally' want to look after the child with a disability, and not wanting them ever to perceive their sibling as a burden.

> I don't want to see them having to curtail their lives because they need to look after Laura. I mean if Alice or Ruth want to go and live in England or Canada or Italy, then I want them to be able to do that. We hope they will care enough about Laura to want to keep an eye on her, but you can't force that. You hear enough about siblings of kids with disabilities to know that they can grow up with a kind of burden of guilt, or worse, a burden of resentment, because they've been required to look after them, or because they've been told so often how lucky they are that they don't have a disability. I don't want Alice or Ruth to feel that kind of burden. Laura is not their responsibility, so Luke and I have to take on board how we are going to look after her. (Jude Lawrence)

Many parents, such as Trish Weston when her family was still young, expressed the belief that having had a sibling with a disability had made their children better people, more compassionate and inclusive, and hoped this would continue in the future.

> I guess our concerns for the girls is how the longer term implications — if Will isn't particularly independent — will affect the way they feel about him, if they feel responsible for him. So that remains to be seen. By and large, I guess they would have been lovely, sensitive, caring little girls anyway, but I think that maybe this has added another dimension to it.

But family featured explicitly in many people's future plans. Carol Lambert was confident that her family would continue to support Malia within the Aboriginal community.

> Cousins and all my nieces and nephews, all the extended family, they look after her. I think they'll look after her, because they're real fond of her now.

Janet Rossi also saw family support as paramount, not least because Sandra herself looked to the family first.

> I mean she's very family orientated, to be taken out of her family environment it would affect her greatly. She's got real principles on those sorts of things.

Similarly, while Sunil Ravi had few concerns about his daughter Amber's capacity to live alone and to support herself independently, with some minor intervention, he believed family would continue to play a role in emotional support.

> I don't know, but it seems to me marriage is not as important as being independent and making a living on her own. She can be alone, in her own world; it's not necessary to have a husband. By the time she gets to that age we'll talk to her

and see if she wants to go on her own. That's fine to me. I don't see any problem. All she needs is her mum or sister, or friends, just to come and talk to her and say hello. She can go to a job, work.

While interviewing for this project, I spoke to three different families where sisters were willingly looking after a brother with Down syndrome, directly or indirectly. However, where people with Down syndrome have no family support as they age, or where siblings cannot or do not wish to take on this role, government-supported community living is a likely eventual outcome. State accommodation is generally made available on the basis of need, with individuals with no family support assessed as having higher needs. Ultimately, people with Down syndrome will be housed somewhere once their families are no longer able to care for them. From the parents' perspective however, the more pressing need is to see their child with a disability develop a secure, viable and enduring system of support before the parents pass on.

The accommodation arrangements of the many people with Down syndrome featured in this book varied from living independently in the community to living at home with their parents. One older man I interviewed lived in his own home with a full-time carer; one couple was married; others lived in group homes. None was in residential care and none had ever been institutionalised.

Trevor Simpson, born in 1943, was one of the earliest people with an intellectual disability such as Down syndrome to live in the community. When he was in his thirties he had the opportunity to go into one of the first houses established by Catholic Care (later identitywa) in Western Australia, and he had the benefit of some essential training before that happened. Mavis Simpson tells the story.

The idea was to prepare people to increase their independence and be able to live more independently and it was quite successful with Trevor. He eventually moved from that house into a Homeswest house which was rented. The three men share the rent and they get it at a special rate, I think, and they seem quite happy there.

Trevor and his two housemates, both of whom also had Down syndrome, needed quite a bit of support, but with appropriate structures in place, he lived there for many years.

The support gradually lessened as they've got more independent, but a social trainer [support worker] comes in nearly every afternoon, Tuesday until Saturday, when they come home from work and stays until about nine o'clock. They're supposed to cook their own meals, but with help. And I don't know that they do a great deal of cooking. I think takeaways do feature somewhat! And then they discuss what they are going to do for the week. What arrangements they are going to make, what shopping they are going to do, and how much money they will need to draw out of their bank accounts to pay their rent and do their shopping and provide for clothes or anything else they want to buy. They have to try and work out whether they've got enough money.

And they do their own housekeeping, their weekly cleaning and washing, but they do have a woman who comes in once a week and she does the cleaning of the floors and that sort of thing. But they keep their rooms as tidy as most lads, I would think, and they do their own ironing and washing and all that. So they're fairly independent. And they all decide what they want to do on the weekend and they talk that over with the supervisor, and the social trainer comes in on Saturdays when they do their washing and ironing — they have set days for doing that, and the days they cook. But if they want to go to the pictures, they can go to the pictures. Two of them can go, perhaps and the other one stays home. They try to encourage them to do things separately, away from the others, you know, go out with other friends or something like that, but they very much seem to want to stick together.

William Mann spoke of Geoffrey's first group home, which was similar to the supervised small group household where Trevor lived.

Geoffrey liked it. But he spent a lot of time here. He'd come home every weekend just about. And eventually they moved him out of his room while we were away once, unbeknown to us, and put him in to share a room with a guy that we didn't want him to be sharing a room with and we started to protest. And they said they'd asked Geoffrey if he was willing to, and of course he said yes to everything. And there was a situation where I think he was beaten up by one of the residents, but we never understood what actually happened and really only pieced it together several years later. But we eventually took him out.

After that initial placement, Geoffrey settled very well into an Activ group home where he and his parents both felt he would stay indefinitely.

He's very happy there. This house is quite different in that it is a mixed home, two ladies and two men, and they had all come from very caring households, and they came into the house as adults. Some of the people that Geoffrey had lived with in the previous group home had been institutionalised since birth and the people he's living with now all have a very caring attitude to each other. They're very supportive, always courteous to each other and the whole atmosphere is quite different, and Geoffrey is learning to regard that as his main home, although he still likes to come home at weekends quite often ...

There's no question that he will always need support. In a house where one staff member has to see to the needs of four or five, he obviously only gets a certain proportion of the staff time but he can cope with that situation. It doesn't distress him and he's quite happy to help with the general chores, you know, go shopping, and help with the meal preparation and washing up and so on. He does his own laundry and ironing. But he'll always need prompting, reminders and assistance; he'll always need guidance. (Muriel Mann)

The assault which his parents feared Geoffrey had experienced in his first group home underlines the difficulties faced by vulnerable people in the community, especially those who are not articulate, and these sorts of issues can feature strongly in a parent's reluctance to pursue supported independent living for their children.

Financial management seemed to be one of the more difficult areas for people living independently, as Trevor's mother Mavis said of him and his mates.

They don't have a concept of the value of money. That seems to be the hardest thing for him to grasp, how you calculate and how you appreciate the value of money and what it will buy. It doesn't worry him. As long as he's got enough money there, he'll get as much as he can.

Muriel Mann made a similar point.

I suppose, to put it crudely, where it's perfectly okay to give Geoffrey twenty dollars and assume that he will spend that reasonably on his outings, his recreational activities, and perhaps a drink, you wouldn't give him two hundred dollars and assume that he'll spend that appropriately.

The Manns saw this in the larger context of the need for carers to be more controlling — more parental perhaps — in financial and other matters, but this was sometimes at odds with the carers' views of their responsibilities towards their clients. William Mann explained that in Geoffrey's first group home, 'they went overboard with the freedoms.'

Whenever we'd go down there one of the guys was walking up to one of the takeaways and buying another meal, even though they had already had one at home, and when we mentioned this to the staff they'd say, 'Well, that's their right. They're living independently,' but I thought it was ridiculous. Geoffrey was doing the same sort of thing, and then when he'd run out of money he'd go to the shop and help himself to things. And it took us a while to discover that this was happening and then having to try and explain to him that this was not done. And once, when he told the social trainer he wanted a drink, he went in and helped himself and came out while the social trainer stayed in the car, and the shopkeeper came out and said, 'I'm sorry, but he didn't pay for that drink.' The worry I have about the future is that in a group home or even at work, he won't be as closely supervised as he is now and that sort of situation could be dangerous, could be quite serious.

An understandable concern was that such behaviour could put vulnerable people at risk with the law. While the proportion of people with intellectual disabilities in the prison system is significantly higher than in the general population, the representation of people with Down syndrome appears to be very much lower than in the population as a whole.[120] Nonetheless the issue of the extent of control or freedom for their adult children is a real one for parents. The 'dignity of risk' — exercising independence in making and learning from your own mistakes — can be a hard concept to embrace when you do so on behalf of someone else. However, as Dirk Bakker put it, 'You can be over-protective; it becomes a limitation, so that they don't live on their own because you try to protect them too much.'

Eloise Hartley and Rachel Kingston have lived independently of their families in their shared apartment since their early twenties. They plan, shop and cook together, and balance their household duties and chores around each other: one day a week each for laundry; a roster for cooking.

> **Eloise**: We take turns at that. We have two days. I do Saturday and Monday and Rachel does Wednesdays and Thursdays. Stir-fry, fish. We get the frozen ones from the shop and then we just put them into the oven. We've been cooking rice, chicken ...
> **Rachel**: I cook a lot of stuff, like I can cook stir-fry as well. I can cook chilli con carne — my favourite.
> **Eloise**: Tuesdays we have a frozen dinner. Then we have Subway on Friday night. We just write down what we want to cook for the week and then we put it on a list and then we'll go down to the shop and get it.

Though their parents visited and kept in close touch (perhaps closer than the two young women recognised or acknowledged), when I interviewed Eloise and Rachel in their home Rachel's parents were away and Eloise's had just returned from an overseas trip. Seemingly their parents pursued 'normal' active lives confident that their adult daughters were able to care for themselves without constant intervention.

Eloise said of her parents, 'I don't get to see them much, because they're always away,' so the young women certainly see themselves as living lives quite separate from their families. They do however get help with their bills; as Eloise said, 'Well, Mum usually helps. I've been trying to add it up myself, but all the hard bits I can't do.' Similarly with the doctor: while their parents were there when needed, Eloise's mother encouraged her independence.

> She told me that I don't have to ask her to come with me any more. If I do feel really sick I do ring Mum, but if I have any other problems I just call the medical centre just down here and then I just go there myself.

Dental appointments were made when the surgery sent reminders about their regular check-ups; a torn nail might mean a trip to the local manicurist for help with filing. They also had someone to come in weekly to assist with the cleaning, though it was recognised as being primarily their own responsibility. Rachel in particular took charge in this area, and had her allocated duties set out on a work sheet.

While the young women have support structures in place, including parents, siblings, and some paid assistance, they are actively self-sufficient. Both have jobs (Rachel one job, Eloise two) to which they travel daily on public transport, and they have the gym, where they work out a couple of times a week with a personal trainer. Their unit, in a complex with front door security, is safe and secure, close to the social facilities and amenities which the young women want, and with excellent public transport connections. They are of course fortunate that one of their families had the financial capacity to enable them to live in such a location. But they are not unique.

I interviewed two other single women, both with Down syndrome, who lived in a unit in Perth which Christine Conway, then in her thirties, was buying herself. She had been able to buy in the 1990s before the price of housing went through the ceiling in Perth; in the early years of the twenty-first century, it is far less likely that any young single woman on a low or even moderate income would be in a position to take out a mortgage, as Christine did, without very significant family support.

Christine and her flatmate Geraldine Howe, in her forties, managed their lives with more support than Eloise and Rachel. They both travelled independently to their part-time jobs in supported employment, and their social lives were centred around disability-based groups such as the Friday Club and the Sunday Club and organised weekend outings to sporting activities, bowling, pubs, movies and occasionally the casino. They also took group holidays with other people with disabilities, to Bali for example. But as Christine said, 'We like to stay home,' where television soaps such as *Neighbours* and *Home and Away* were an important part of their fairly structured daily routine.

Christine had previously lived in her family home and she retained a lot of contact with her parents, who visited very frequently; Geraldine lost her parents when she was much younger and had been living in a hostel for many years before moving in with Christine, but she did have some continuing contact with siblings. The women had a support worker who visited them regularly and helped with things such as organising their medication regime, by putting their daily tablets into pill boxes. She would also make arrangements for them to visit doctors if necessary, the hairdresser or the dentist, or perhaps Christine would phone her mother if she or Geraldine were ill.

Rather than a written shopping list, the women prepared a list of their household needs based on Compic pictographs,[121] simple images of groceries and household items, and their carer would drive them home with their groceries after their weekly shopping excursion. The women shared the cooking, which largely consisted of dishes such as salads, fish fingers, spaghetti bolognaise, chicken and a weekly takeaway, and took joint responsibility for cleaning and laundry. Unfortunately, some time after I interviewed Christine and Geraldine, their shared housing arrangement fell through. Geraldine moved elsewhere and Christine rented out her unit and subsequently returned home to live with her family, though she continued looking for another flatmate.

Another young man who lived alone with even less support than Rachel and Eloise was Jeremy Young. In his late twenties at the time I first spoke to him, Jeremy was very proud of his independence, his unit and his lifestyle. The day I met him at his home, his mother had dropped by to witness his signature on a change of electoral enrolment. Although she was a regular visitor to her son's home, on the whole he managed without her keeping more than a cursory maternal eye on proceedings.

> I used to have a social trainer, but I don't see her anymore. My mum comes down to see how everything goes and if there are any problems or anything.

If he needed to see a doctor or a dentist or get a haircut, he made his own appointments. He also managed his own bills with his bankcard: 'electricity bills, water bills and some Telstra bills and my mobile phone bill. Sometimes I have help, sometimes they are automatically paid' from the bank account into which his salary and his supplementary pension were both paid. Though Jeremy suggested he sometimes had trouble with his budget, his attitude to money was very careful.

Jeremy: I do my own shopping. Once a fortnight. I do grocery shopping in the supermarket and do my vegie shopping at the markets, because they're cheaper that way.

I like using money. I tend to sometimes overspend a bit, and that's a bit of a problem really! My mum's trying to help me to get onto a budget, and it's been okay. It's been a little bit up and down. So, I'm learning how to save, which I have been ...

And I do love it here because it is so central, it's just that the rent I am paying is not just for the apartment, it's also for a parking bay that's supplied.

Jan: Which you don't use?

Jeremy: No, only for visitors, because I don't drive — one day I might. I am kind of worried about my rent, because it is too much and I would like to find somewhere that has lower rent; or not rent at all!

Jeremy's transition to independent living was facilitated by spending time in a caravan at his family home, where he learned the important step of enjoying his own company. He'd also taken practical steps such as learning to cook. But still, moving out for him 'was a very big step.'

Because I have diabetes, and having diabetes and living on my own was a very big step in my life — which I am happy about. Because, when I first had diabetes, my mum helped me to eat well and made sure I had the things to go by, because I couldn't understand about diabetes when I first had it. And I do have regular check-ups as well at the Fremantle Hospital. And so it was a very big step for me which I am very proud of, living on my own, with diabetes, and because some people when they have diabetes, they sometimes they are very scared of living on their own and I just felt that it was time for me to move on and — so here I am.

For Jeremy, having diabetes was a much more significant obstacle to independent living than the fact that he had Down syndrome. Though proud of his capacity to live independently, Jeremy had also thought about sharing.

Jeremy: I did that once, you know, when I used to live in Perth. And that was okay. And, now I am here in my own apartment, which is fine; but I don't see myself here in generations to come now. I see myself moving in with someone.
Jan: You would prefer that?
Jeremy: Yes.
Jan: For friendship.
Jeremy: Friendship, or the other.
Jan: Relationship, yes?
Jeremy: Yes.

Jeremy subsequently moved into a different unit in the suburbs, but he still lives by himself, and acknowledged that he was quite often lonely.

Ellen Wentworth and Adam Szabo, who both have Down syndrome, got married in 2009 when Ellen was thirty-seven and Adam was forty. The two met each other through a Citizen Advocacy group in the south-west town where they now live and for a while it was a long-distance relationship because Adam lived out of town. Once it became clear it was serious, Ellen's parents settled on finding the unit where the couple would eventually live. Ellen was still living at home at this stage, where her mother Leah described her as her 'star boarder'. In the family home Ellen had developed excellent housekeeping skills. As well, she has had a part-time job at a local fast food outlet since she was seventeen, and another job in a cafe cleaning tables and serving, so she was already competent to manage a household. Ellen moved into the unit by herself and though she said that at first 'I missed my parents,' she enjoyed her independence.

Once the two were officially engaged in January 2006, Adam moved in.

For practical reasons, Leah would have preferred Adam to have had some experience living independently before moving in with Ellen. He had been the last child living at home with his mother after his elder siblings moved out, and Leah was concerned that, with Ellen's experience in housekeeping, she might end up taking over a mothering role — not an unusual occurrence in marriages when young men move straight out of home. But Adam has learned a great deal since they have been living together and there is a fairly strict division of work within the household. They share different aspects of cleaning their unit: Adam washes up and prepares breakfast; Ellen cooks dinner. Her repertoire includes grilled chops and steak, meatballs, chicken in soy sauce, stir-fry and lots of vegetables.

Adam thought it was right for them to be married and so did his mother. As he said, 'It's fine with her and as long as she is happy I am happy as well.' He also said, 'I think it's great because we are the last ones.' As far as he was concerned, all their siblings were married, so it was appropriate that he and Ellen got married as well. Ellen's parents were happy too and she remembered her father saying to Adam at the wedding: 'Look after our girl.'

The couple leads a very normal life; in fact when I met them I felt quite overwhelmed with the normality of it all — but why shouldn't it be? When I visited their unit one Saturday morning they had just come back from voting at the federal election and were unpacking the shopping and thinking about the birthday party they were holding that evening for Adam. Leah was there too. She takes them shopping every Saturday and then they sit down together to do the weekly budget. Otherwise they need no help, though Ellen felt they would continue to need assistance with financial management. At this Saturday morning session they also make their taxi bookings for the week's recreational activities, though they use public transport — a bus into town then another one out again — to get to their various workplaces. Adam and Ellen will phone Leah for occasional help with transport during the week, but 'It's a request,' Leah says, 'not an expectation.'

Social activities include a bus trip to Perth once a fortnight during the football season with the local supporters' group (they are dedicated West Coast Eagles fans), tenpin bowling and ballroom dancing. Ellen has completed dance medals at the highest level, with gold medals in all styles, and Adam has taken up dancing since meeting her, largely because he wants to be good enough to partner her. Adam also has a strong religious commitment, having served as an altar boy, and he also 'plays the guitar and sings holy songs.' Ellen plays guitar and piano.

Beyond Leah's weekly shopping and budget session, the couple are self-sufficient. Adam receives some support through an employment agency for his job at Woolworths (Ellen is unsupported and on a full wage in both her jobs), but otherwise they do not use any government services. However Leah recognises that the extended family will one day need to take on the supervisory role she presently fills. In the meantime she feels confident leaving Ellen and Adam, sometimes for weeks at a time, with others filling the gap when she travels.

Travel is an important part of Ellen's and Adam's lives too. They have been to Bali with a friend and spent three weeks in New Zealand with Leah. On their honeymoon they toured to Sydney and Melbourne, saw a performance by André Rieu, and travelled back via the Great Ocean Road. Adam, who speaks and writes two languages, corresponds with relatives in Germany and eastern Europe and is keen to take his wife to visit them. So they have a savings fund and each week they note how their money is growing. Such is their dedication to seeing their funds rise that they now pack their own lunches to take to work or recreational outings in order to save money on takeaways.

When I asked if they had thought about having children, both agreed that it was not part of their plans: 'too much work' was the consensus. Ellen takes the contraceptive pill.

What did having Down syndrome mean to this couple? 'Nothing,' said Ellen. That was the way Ellen was brought up, Leah commented; and while Adam's mother, whom he described as 'over-protective because I am the last one,' may have been less demanding of him because of his disability, both Ellen and Adam live a normal everyday life untouched by disability. It's different in one respect though — they don't fight.

At the age of forty-eight, Richard Stevens lives with his full-time live-in carer Gordon Griffith in a small fishing town north of Perth, an idyllic location in many ways.

It's like a little hamlet where the local farmers have holiday homes and places like that. They've got a nice little place right on the water and fish and crayfish and all of those good things, and have a boat. (Jill Mather)

While that situation has been working well for Richie, the prospect of his moving into a group home or sharing his home with other people with disabilities has also been discussed. Gordon and the coordinator at the local community living organisation were testing the water by inviting other individuals involved in the community living group to visit Richie for weekends on a reciprocal basis, with a view to fostering ongoing friendships. The route towards living in a group home in a larger Mid West town, however, was by no means straightforward.

His sister Jill described Richie as 'physically extremely competent. Very competent with housework, very systematic about what had to be done, and when, and in what sequence.' These sorts of skills meant that Richie had learned to drive and though he didn't have a full licence, 'the local police were very helpful and had arranged for Rich to have a special licence that allows him to drive' in his own neighbourhood. But Richie had also developed some very fixed habits, perhaps from sharing a household for a number of years with his father who had emerging Alzheimer's. Richie's emphasis on patterns and sequence, for example, could become compulsive — 'If you happened to be standing on the spot of floor that's due to be vacuumed, you had to move' — and Jill was aware that her brother did not cope well with change.

Richie's parents were loving and caring but had limited expectations about his abilities, a reasonably typical attitude towards people with Down syndrome when Richie was born in the early 1960s, and they had never attempted to prepare him for independent living. From Gordon's point of view, Richie had been over-indulged, and had not been given the opportunity to develop some of the skills which are a usual and necessary part of maturity.

Put it this way, if somebody had have got to him twenty years ago, twenty-five years ago, Richie would be totally independent, maybe just having somebody dropping in, somebody there that he could ring up. Rich won't ring people up on the phone. I know he can do it, he just doesn't do it. It gets back to decision-making. Richie has learnt not to make any decisions because decisions have been made for him all his life. Because if you've got someone there to make a decision for you, why worry about it? (Gordon Griffith)

Consequently, Gordon believed that Richie would find the transition to a situation where he was less fully supported, perhaps in a shared household, a challenge. From a lifetime of having things done 'his way' and for his benefit, Richie had developed habits of dependence so deeply ingrained that he found it hard to accept change. Nor had he been required to accommodate other people's points of view.

There hasn't been expectations put on him that he align himself with the rest of the world; the rest of the world has pretty much shaped itself around him as far as possible. There was never any disciplined kind of statement of, 'You need to learn, you need to do this.' (Jill Mather)

The situation highlights the difficulties of preparing an older person who has always lived with their parents or who has always been cared for, for a less supported environment. Waiting until a time of critical need arises may be waiting too long, as Anna Klein said of her son Michael.

You have all these years when they are young and teenagers, 'Oh it's all right, I don't have to worry about that just now.' But I'm going to be sixty this year and he's twenty-four, going on twenty-five, so it's time for him to move on somewhere. I don't want to wait until I'm not able to do it any more because then, panic sets in and I want him to be comfortable by that time.

For Richie, a move to a different locality would also mean severing deep roots in his local community.

> He's got a massive friendship recognition place here. As well as that, the locals would most probably freak! They really do, without Richie there they don't know what to do sometimes. People love Richie, we're continually getting things like, 'How's Richie going?' and all that. (Gordon Griffith)

Yet Jill also felt that Richie was not treated as an adult by the people of the town, that there was 'an assumption on the part of the community that he's a perpetual child, and there's been no kind of appropriate ageing into social behaviour.' His parents had treated him the same way. Consequently he was not invited to socialise in the local community in ways which she would have liked and which she believed would have been beneficial for him.

Richie's situation illustrates the need to work actively at developing appropriate community relationships, and indeed, creating community networks is now a major strategy in developing independent living for people with disabilities. In the right circumstances though, active community inclusion of a person with disability can sometimes emerge spontaneously. Wendy Brookton described what some would consider virtually a model for setting up community support, as something which could easily develop in a rural community with only a little bit of initiative required.

> Look, I would try and pick out the people involved in someone's life and just throw the issues around. Say, okay, well you know, what are the issues? Mark, what are you feeling like you're missing out on? What do you want to do? If you can't achieve it yet, how are you going to achieve it? Throw it around and someone's going to come up with

an answer. Get a heap of brains in there and work it out. People go, oh yes; oh we'll do that. Getting that sort of thing happening, I actually don't think it's as hard as what people think it's going to be. Really I don't think it's that difficult to do. It's just a matter of saying, righty-o, we're going to do this and then following it through and getting other people to follow it through.

Charlie King has always been supported by his local community in the small town where he lives in the north of the state. His extended Aboriginal family — siblings, cousins, aunties and uncles — involves a broader family network than does most non-Indigenous families, and this network serves exactly the purpose that many city-based nuclear families are presently trying to achieve for their family member with a disability. Charlie is very well known within his community and as his sister Rhonda Henry said of his informal network of friends: 'If they take Charlie out, they protect him. If anybody tries to do something out of the ordinary, they all gang up on them.'

Marg King: Like for example, he went out to the pub one night and a few guys had come into town. Charlie was standing up near the speakers because he loves music — music is magic when it comes to Charlie, eh? — and these guys started rough-handling him. They got thrown out in the end, they had six other guys on top of them and this is not just the local Aboriginal boys; a couple of the white guys were involved in it, they all knew Charlie. So those two guys got kicked out of the pub.

Jan: So the whole community looks out for him?

Rhonda Henry: Yeah. And we had one incident where this fellow from Halls Creek or something, at the pub one night he was asking for a cigarette. Charlie's very canny when it comes to his smokes, he won't part with them. He turned around and told this guy, 'No, I don't have any.' This guy kept pestering him. Charlie just told him, 'Look, go away.' This guy punched him in the stomach and winded him. But the other guys that were there saw it all happening, and they got stuck into this bloke. So he left town. Apparently people had heard from Wyndham all the way up to Kununurra, all the way up to Broome about what had happened to Charlie, and they told this guy, 'If you come to this town, we'll be after you!' Anywhere Charlie goes people will look after him, he's popular around people. Everyone basically knows who he is and if somebody just steps out of line with him, he's got all these people around him to help him out.

The only real safety concern was Charlie's poor vision and because of that, his sisters kept a close watch on his movements at night.

We give him limited time to come home; if he's not home by nine, ten o'clock at night, we'll just ring around, or go check. One of the boys will always say, 'No, no, he's all right, we'll bring him home.'

One interesting aspect of Charlie's social network is that his group of friends gets younger and younger as Charlie ages. As the young men in the town move on, or become more immersed in their own family lives, others automatically take their place, so while the level of community support is constant, the individuals who play a role in Charlie's life change.

Another man of similar age to Charlie, and also from an extended Aboriginal family, has experienced very different circumstances. Frank Flynn (born 1969) lives in another small town in the Kimberley with his older sister. His mother was the daughter of two members of the stolen generations who were brought up together at Forrest River mission and who married there. But though she herself had a large family, circumstances have meant that there is only limited support for Frank from his siblings. Because of the absence of facilities for Frank in the Kimberley in the 1970s, Frank's mother moved south with him to enable him to attend special schools. On completing high school he got work in an Activ workshop while his mother returned to the north with a view to settling Frank into the community in his own home.

When Frank's mother passed on some eight years after their return from down south, his care and responsibility devolved completely onto his eldest sister Denise. Frank developed health problems, including diabetes, and he and Denise went back down to Perth for his health and her employment. There he spent a number of years before returning once again to the north but, as Denise said, 'He was too unwell for any employment. It's taken him two to three years to just get healthy again.'

Frank's extended absences from his family have disrupted the development of the kind of kinship network within the Aboriginal community which has spontaneously grown up around Charlie. This was not an unusual situation, as Eddie Bartnik from Disability Services Commission acknowledged.

The other thing that we found particularly distressing. Aboriginal children from the north-west would often come to Perth for medical treatment and then they'd often find their way into respite facilities and some of them never returned home. So there were people being separated from their families and communities.

And for both these men living in the Kimberley, there are virtually no services available except for Home and

Community Care (HACC) and residences for the elderly. In the absence of both state services and a strong network of family support, Denise Flynn believes it is inevitable that Frank will end up in an aged-care facility. Until that happens though, he continues to live with her.

For most people, the prospect of outliving their child with a disability is unrealistic, but they usually have time to prepare for the certainty of their own death. Penny Innes had less time than most. The sole parent of an only child, she died a short time after I interviewed her when her daughter Rebecca was just twenty. Though she faced the prospect of her imminent death with great anxiety on Rebecca's account, she had prepared her daughter for an independent life from her earliest years. Rebecca grew up with a mother who held the highest expectations for her. She had an inclusive education in a small town outside Perth, and she and her mother were actively involved in a parent-based educational organisation which helped Penny access learning materials and educational strategies to complement Rebecca's school-based education.

Rebecca now lives on her own in the town where she grew up, where she is supported through a private support agency under a system planned by her mother before her death. She has guardians, a financial trustee, and is learning to live independently through the help of support workers and her local area coordinator, whose role has become one of friend.

How it works is I have a disability pension, and I get some funding from my disability fund, and it gives me funding for a support agency. The specific reason was for me to have support with them because my mum passed away and they came in and just took over Mum's role. That was the position, to take over my mum's role and to help me with my independence, because my mum wasn't there to support me. My mum set everything up for me.

After her mother died, Rebecca moved from the home they had shared a little way out of town into a comfortable unit she owns in town itself. As Rebecca said, she is better situated there, especially with regard to transport because in her former home, 'I didn't have anything. I was stranded out there. I was isolated.' This unit is reasonably close to the beach, shops and public transport.

There are three bedrooms. One is my yoga, spiritual room, I would say. The second bedroom is mine and the third bedroom is the spare bedroom, like you have a flatmate in. There is a bathroom and a toilet and there's the laundry. A lounge room, a dining room and a kitchen. It's a duplex.

Rebecca describes herself as 'independent in my unit.' She sustains this independence with the help of support agency staff, who facilitate social and recreation activities, assist with shopping and help her prepare her menus. Rebecca maintains the vegetarian diet she learned from her mother as well, cooking 'vegetarian pizzas, pasta. Lots of salad, salad wraps, mixed salads. Roast vegetables, I cook a whole lot.' While Rebecca is still in the early stages of the transition to independence, agency staff sleep over several nights a week.

Not every single night; some nights I'm independent. I am independent on Tuesday night and Thursday nights.

Though she is still finding some aspects of living alone a challenge, Rebecca is determined to follow in her mother's path, pursuing her interests in yoga, dance, art and spirituality. She has a strong network of support in the area where she lives, and is well known in the community. With most of her friends tending to be older people she has met through her support agency or through her mother's connections,

Rebecca is also working on developing a group of friends her own age. At the time of our second interview, she was still struggling with the impact of her bereavement but as time passes, particularly once she finds a continuing job or study opportunities, she is hopeful that new friendships will give her greater access to the 'coffees, night clubs, bowling' activities she enjoys.

Finding accommodation is not always straightforward, even though there is now more support available as the notion of inclusion is promoted through community and government agencies. Funding and the availability of places does not match demand, which has been a point of contention for successive state governments. Bernard Grant spoke about the continuing struggle he and his wife Angela had gone through with Disability Services Commission to find some form of independent living for his son Angus. To facilitate this, the family first had to apply for government support.

You apply through a provider. We chose Catholic Care because we felt they had a commitment to the long-term care of our child, so we went through this process with them. Then they presented the application to Disability Services ...

It's all quite a harrowing experience. We came out of the interview emotionally drenched because you have to come up with the worst scenarios you can imagine for him to go into care. Basically, they want you to prove that his behaviour is at risk to himself or at risk to someone in the family, serious risk. So to prove that you have to say some pretty dreadful things. Well obviously we haven't convinced anybody that that's the case. We originally put in for it more than ten years ago but the results come back and we're still in the bottom rung. There's three different rungs. You either get the funding, or you're next in line, or else you're not in dire need.

That was in August 2008. A year later, the story was different —finally the family had been offered accommodation support funding.

This covered staffing costs for the care of Angus with the provider of our choice in the community outside the family home. The funding does not include personal needs such as clothing, transport, medical needs and social outings etc, only the essentials of living.

The family was elated, but more than fifteen years had gone by since they first applied.

Once funding is made available, the family and individual can consider different options: a place in a group home like Geoffrey Mann, or supported accommodation with a carer in one's own home like Richie, or a Homeswest (now Department of Housing) home like Trevor Simpson. The Grants are opting for a private service provider. But first of all, you have to get the funding.

Just as people once fought against the institutionalisation of their children in the early years of their lives, most parents of younger people with Down syndrome react against any prospect of having their children institutionalised or placed in state care. For carers of older people with Down syndrome though, facing the prospect of finding long-term care for those who have not developed the skills for independent living, it's sometimes hard to contemplate alternatives to some form of institutionalised living. Even accommodation in an aged care facility might seem an appropriate, even a positively beneficial placement. It was an option Jill Mather considered for Richie when their mother went into full-time care.

The woman who was the manager at the home when Mum first moved there actually talked blithely about the possibility of Rich being able to live there with them. But when I went through people at the Department of Ageing about the criteria and what have you, they said, 'Oh absolutely not, it would be socially inappropriate; he's a young man, he needs to be with young people.' I said, 'I'm sorry but we're talking about someone who's lived with my parents and the people that he socialises with are of that age group for the most part, have been all his life.' We're not talking about someone who's out here, young and twenties and going to discos and clubbing who suddenly gets lobbed into an aged care facility. When it comes to the issue of Downs people ageing, try talking to the Department of Ageing and say, 'What's your profile for where aged Downs people can go?' And they don't have one.

Sadly, there is a logic to Jill's argument — if people with Down syndrome stay at home as their parents age, and don't mix with other people of their own age, then their social lives will tend to centre on older people, however inappropriate that might appear to others.

Denise Flynn shared Jill's view. When Denise and her brother Frank returned to the Kimberley after some years down south she found suitable support facilities for Frank very limited. Because of his temperament and personal history, she believed he would be better off and happier in a facility for older people than in one for people with generic disabilities.

He's not old, but he's always mixed with the oldies anyway, so they're no problem for him to mix with. I mean he's not getting any younger and he does have all sorts of problems. He wouldn't be able to be in a place with handicapped people because he gets frightened of them, like when they break out and get angry. Because that's what happened when he was going on outings down in Perth, some of the guys were getting angry and he got quite frightened of that.

But in their small Kimberley community, there was little chance of her brother finding a place in any facility, whether for the aged or for the people with disabilities.

In Perth they've got private facilities for the elderly, which means semi-supported accommodation, where you've got units, but you've also got a central day care, and you've got central eating facilities. I see that as absolutely ideal. But I don't think they've got anything like that for the disabled.

Another Kimberley family found aged care facilities a poor solution for their respite needs, though it was the only one available.

If I want to go away I can book Sandra into the Aged Care Centre. They have units and they have someone there caretaking it. You've got to book in advance to get a place in there. That's okay, but it's more designed for the old people. She used to go there and do activities with the elderly people a while ago, but it wasn't stimulating enough. She just kept saying, 'It's not my thing, I don't want to be here.' (Janet Rossi)

In the 1990s, at least one regional family support group attempted to set up supported accommodation such as Denise wanted for Frank but, as Janet Rossi recalled, the attempt was unsuccessful, as the group's idea of supported residential accommodation was at odds with government initiatives on community-based inclusion.

I'd have peace of mind if Sandra was in a controlled sort of place where they can live independently in their own units and have carers come in and check on them, have someone there that can monitor who comes and goes. Some security more than anything. I think most of the parents felt like that at the time and wanted something done, but the guy from Disability Services wasn't very supportive. He more or less termed it as putting them into a ghetto again and you see now how the government's trying to streamline them into normal society, so the thing fell apart. It got away from what most parents wanted and now the thing's just folded.

On the other hand, some things became possible in country areas which would perhaps not have been contemplated in Perth. Charlie King's sisters knew exactly what they wanted for him. While not a permanent or even perhaps a long-term solution, it certainly met Charlie's needs for a while.

Rhonda Henry: I got support off Disability Services to purchase a caravan a few years back for Charlie. In that sense it was quite good, because he moves around. They said, 'Oh you should get him a house,' and we said, 'We don't want a house.'

Mary King: Yes, if he had a house he wouldn't …

Rhonda: He wouldn't stay in there anyway.

Jan: How would you have got a house?

Rhonda: You probably could get one through Homeswest, a house or a flat. Renting.

Jan: Here?

Mary: It could be anywhere really, wherever …

Rhonda: Depending on where he is, yes.

Mary: Well, Charlie doesn't stay put for long, so …

Rhonda: The caravan moves from place to place; where Charlie went, the caravan went. Then the caravan sort of fell to bits and we ended up having him back in a room.

One of the newer accommodation possibilities in Perth for people with disabilities is purpose-built cluster housing. Amelia Bakker and Alex Major are both hoping to go into the second of two new complexes being developed in Perth's western suburbs. The Bakker family's long-term plan was to have their daughter Amelia living independently by the time she was twenty-five or thirty.

> We thought, all right, shall we buy a unit or rent a unit? But then she would be isolated and we heard from others that really that's the main problem they have; if they get housing from DHW,[122] then they're isolated, even if people come to them to go out or to do things, they're still isolated. (Dirk Bakker)

In 2002 the family heard of the first housing project where a cluster of two-bedroom apartments had been built for people with disabilities on land in an attractive local suburb, in a cooperative venture facilitated by the local council, DSC and highly committed parents. The parent planning group that the Bakkers subsequently joined however, decided that one element was missing from the original concept.

> It's fairly well set up, it blends in very well, and everybody's very happy there. Then they found that still they didn't mix, that the kids do their work, they come home, but still they stay on their own. So now they've started, once a month, a get-together in one of the apartments, and that works very well. (Dirk Bakker)

Keeping the idea of creating a community within the community as well as linking to the larger community,[123] the second housing project group — comprising parents and a number of people with Down syndrome as well as people with other disabilities whose support needs ranged from low to moderately high — decided to adopt a slightly different approach in their planning. They designed a cluster housing complex of six two-bedroom apartments located around a house that comprised four one-bedroom units, each with its own bathroom and some with cooking facilities, and a large kitchen and family area. This living area would be the heart of the complex and accessible to all the residents. One of the self-contained one-bedroom units would be designated for a live-in carer.

They found land for the complex located in an area of social housing and the parents envisaged that the structure of the complex would facilitate social interaction, both within the complex and with the surrounding community.

> We'll try to do regular interactions on a monthly basis, or quarterly basis, with the people who live on the same block, and then the people from the neighbourhood, so we have three different levels of social interaction. And we will try to get some kind of facilitator in to do that. So the principle is that they live on their own, they do their own thing, and then maybe once a week they get together with the people that they live with. And whenever they come home they can always go to that central meeting point. So if they want to socialise, they can. (Dirk Bakker)

The Department of Housing (DHW or Homeswest) would build and own the complex and the local council would own the land but would be recompensed for its use. The residents would be Homeswest tenants and as such would pay a subsidised weekly rent.

> In principle our kids are very low on the DHW housing list — until we are half dead or crippled we are very low on the list — but because we do this with a group, because we put

quite a bit of effort in to get the land, we think we should have the right to live in it. (Dirk Bakker)

The scheme has involved a number of committed families working together for over a decade to bring it to fruition, and is likely to involve continuing parental support for quite some time. Planning has also entailed forging a friendship group among the prospective residents, who have been involved in the planning meetings and associated social functions over many years. For some, like Dirk's daughter Amelia, the plan to move them out of the family home took some getting used to.

Amelia comes to the meetings, and certainly we're trying to get her involved. She is now reasonably used to it and she asks about it, but certainly the first year, she was very hesitant. She was concerned that she would be left on her own basically, that she would live on her own without support. We said, 'No, there's no way.'

A feature of the project was that each member of the group would have the benefit of an external support group established to support their ongoing needs. Dirk Bakker was adamant that the system had to be self-sustaining, that the parents would be in a position where ultimately they could back away.

Probably more critical than the housing and the land etc., is how they do it when we are not here. Basically we found it must be, what they say, self-sustainable; that if we are not there it still runs. So that's probably the challenge.

A formal supervisory system such as a microboard was essential for each individual in the group, to provide some form of 'governance': a team of people to take continuing responsibility for the residents for their lifetime, for the management of what Dirk called 'life issues'.

They set up a group of maybe three, four people, that have an interest in the child and have regular meetings, maybe once a month or so, to see how the child is going and what adjustments are needed with the child. That's officially set up. Sometimes, yes, a family member can get involved, but most of them try initially to do without, or maybe with just one family member as part of the small group. So that's what they call the microboard.

This housing group has been working on this project for nearly a decade, and in 2010 it still seemed as if it would not be open for business until at least 2012.

Opportunities for the sort of group living enjoyed by Geoffrey and Trevor or the housing cooperative which the Bakker family are working towards, are certainly more limited outside Perth but there are some innovative accommodation schemes emerging in regional centres. The Mid West Community Living Association (MWCLA) in Geraldton, a town about four hundred kilometres north of Perth, is a non-government organisation part-funded by Disability Services Commission, but its origins recall many other services which developed because of personal or private initiative. It emerged just a few years ago when, in response to the needs of one individual, a family group set in place a system of supported accommodation. By 2010, MWCLA provided ongoing accommodation support for about twenty individuals with disabilities living in the Mid West area, including some with Down syndrome. Support varies according the needs of the individual. 'Good neighbours' living close at hand might offer daily support for cooking, evening company, or assistance with bills and paperwork, in return for subsidised rent; live-in carers offer more intensive support. Some individuals live independently but have an occasional support person drop in to ensure everything is going well, or perhaps to act as a buffer in dealings with public and private organisations: for example, facilitating arrangements with Centrelink, or with the Department of Housing and Works (Homeswest) which, through its community housing program, provides most of the accommodation available through MWCLA. As well as meeting the regular daily needs of the people it supports, MWCLA also acts as a means of facilitating community interaction, through occasional picnics, barbecues, outings and get-togethers, and by making and supporting connections for individuals within their local area.[124]

The structured community interaction incorporated into the cluster housing project or organisations such as MWCLA is fundamental to current understandings of the living needs of people with disabilities in Western Australia where, in a move increasingly facilitated by the state through Disability Services Commission, the focus is shifting towards establishing networks that support people living in a community rather than simply providing the physical bricks and mortar to house them. This policy is embedded in DSC's Community Living Initiative launched in 2008.

> It aims to establish a broader range of alternative community living arrangements for adults, which are sustainable, culturally appropriate and outside the traditional models of accommodation. Each community living arrangement is 'person-centred' and emphasises key elements of a 'home' in the community and 'a good life' such as valued relationships, choice, contribution, security for the future and challenge.[125]

In addition, a number of non-government self-help organisations with similar philosophies have emerged in Western Australia, often modelled on institutions elsewhere.

One is the Planned Individual Network (PIN), which draws directly on a pioneering Canadian model known as PLAN.[126] The emphasis of PIN is on creating independence through personal networks in social rather than physical structures,[127] and the Grant family saw their membership of the organisation as 'a concerted, directed effort at organising the future for Angus and making sure that he has people around him who have his interests at heart.'

> The whole idea of PIN is, people's quality of life is related to the quality of relationships you have. You can't just say, well he's got housing so you can wash your hands of it, and he'll be all right. Their quality of life, as anybody's does, relates to having relationships. So the idea with PIN is to try to set up a network of people so that should you get run over by a bus tomorrow, there'd be people who relate to Angus, who understand him and value him. It's a two-way relationship, an ongoing relationship, it would be there for him. So we've just started on that. (Bernard Grant)

There is little doubt that social isolation can be a problem for people with disabilities such as Down syndrome who live in the community. Ironically, those who are most able to manage with little support and are therefore least likely to mould their lives around disability-related organisations and support groups, may be the most vulnerable. Helen Golding, for instance, had faith in her daughter Charlotte's capacity to look after herself, perhaps holding down a regular job and managing on a day-to-day level with minimum intervention, but she still had concerns about her being isolated in the community.

> I would prefer that she was living as a part of a group of people at least within walking distance, who she could have

as friends. To be able to network with them and do things socially, not to be totally isolated and everyone saying, 'Isn't that wonderful, she is independent,' because that is not what life is about.

Simple matters like reluctance to use public transport at night and not having a driving licence can lead to social isolation for people living independently, particularly women. Eloise and Rachel for example, though certainly not socially isolated, were limited in their social circle, although they also seemed perfectly happy with it.

Jan: Do the two of you go out together most of the time?
Eloise: Yes, yes, we hang out together all the time.
Jan: What about other friends, do you have people visit sometimes?
Eloise: Well they haven't been coming over that much, because Rachel and I don't have many friends, so that's why we've been going to the gym, get to know the people there. Then I met some people from this film course that I did, and I got their numbers.
Jan: What about you Rachel, do you mainly hang out with Eloise?
Rachel: Oh yes, Eloise is great.
Eloise: Yes, but I am the only friend that you have.
Rachel: Yes, that's true.

Increasingly, online social networking sites such as Facebook are proving tremendously popular with young people with Down syndrome and, even for those with less well developed literacy skills, can create a sense of belonging and be a significant source of valuable social support.

Jeremy, an extremely self-aware and philosophical man and very proud of his independence, was also forthcoming about the downside of living by himself.

Jeremy: I do feel lonely a bit, you know, kind of like wishing I had someone to talk to at night sometimes, but sometimes I do talk to my neighbours a bit, which is good, which is okay. But with me, sometimes I talk to myself, and I don't know why I do it, but it's just a part of life. But I do try *not* to talk to myself too much. It's just sometimes I feel a little a bit lonely, but I don't feel lonely all the time. It's only sometimes. But what I'm doing is trying to get used to having ups and downs ...

Jan: Generally, are you more up or more down?

Jeremy: I get happy. I do get happy. In my life, when there is something going okay and everything is fine, I tend to be happy. And I am trying not to let depression get the best of me, because that's not like me at all. I don't see my life being depressed, I see my life full of happiness and being around nice people.

In many ways the process of community inclusion can be like the process of educational 'mainstreaming'. Being located in a regular classroom does not necessarily mean being part of that classroom, and can mean no more than being 'main-dumped'. Social isolation can sometimes be an outcome, and the experience of people coming out of large institutions such as Kew Cottages in Victoria in the 1990s has shown that living in the community can, ironically, lead to a decline in meaningful social contact for the individual concerned.[128] These sorts of issues underpin the present emphasis on establishing and maintaining continuing social networks for people with disabilities.

Finally, how did parents feel when the nest was a little emptier?

Well it certainly was extraordinary to us, the first few weeks, to find that we were now free, as it were, to accept invitations to go out, go to the theatre or go to a concert, and not always have the complication of wondering whether it was appropriate to get a sitter in or not, or whether Geoffrey could cope on his own. (Muriel Mann)

But the sense of liberation could be 'bitter-sweet' too.

Caring for Angus has dominated our lives for nearly thirty-eight years. Although logic says that eventually, Angus would have to go into supported accommodation outside the family home, how could I as a good parent force him out of his own home, possibly even against his will? He cannot tell us how he feels or tell us what he wants. He won't understand what is happening. Why should he have to move out? Are we just plain selfish or are we doing the right thing in preparing him for a sustainable future without us? Lacking the verbal and personal care skills to fend for himself makes him too vulnerable to live by himself in the community and long term he would have to go into some form of supported accommodation. Nevertheless, the future for us without Angus will take quite some adjustment. I will miss his sense of humour, his enjoyment of the simple things in life, his helpfulness and affection. (Bernard Grant)

In our family, we already have in mind a place where Maddie will live — she has nominated the age of twenty-five as the moment when she will leave us — but we face the prospect with dread, to the point where her father is already teasing her that we might have to move in with her so we don't get too lonely. Jokes aside, we will miss her enormously.

Successful independent living for people with disabilities such as Down syndrome is based on inclusion. Community inclusion means more than just living outside an institution. It requires structures and support in place to facilitate socially based activities and a sense of belonging. But, whether it's social or educational, inclusion has to be supported: it does not just happen. There is still not enough money, not enough support and not enough appropriate housing. To date, families such as the Grants, individuals such as Angus, have had to wait too long. People like Richie Stevens who might have been able to learn to live with less support in a community-based setting if they had had the opportunity to do so earlier, have probably lost the chance to develop skills and independence. There is however increasing government recognition that more needs to be done and that establishing community support structures is as important as the provision of housing itself.

The families of younger people with Down syndrome and with other disabilities are in a better position now to pursue the dream of their family member living 'a good life', knowing that there are many pioneers who are living independently, that there are many different models of community-based living, that there is some real possibility of finetuning choices according to the needs of the person involved, and that there may be some government support available to help facilitate this. The very notion of independent community living is becoming more subtle too. Independent living is not just about living without support — in fact for people with disabilities such as Down syndrome it is highly likely to involve some degree of continuing monitoring and intervention — but living in a way that involves meaningful community interaction and that is 'sustainable' in the longer term. Little if any of this was true for earlier generations of people with Down syndrome and their families.

Building granny flats and buying units; finding places through service providers in supported accommodation; developing long-term shared living strategies with like-minded friends; establishing community networks, microboards and circles of friends: all of these approaches represent a shift away from the philosophy once endorsed by organisations such as the Slow Learning Children's Group in Western Australia, of establishing farm colonies in isolated settings where people with intellectual disabilities could live in peaceful, productive and safe seclusion. The distance between 1950s seclusion and twenty-first century community immersion is immeasurable, with the possibilities available today unimaginable to the members of the SLCG who in the 1950s wondered what on earth was going to happen to their children. Nonetheless the cautious optimism we can dare to feel today is at least partly a legacy of their commitment.

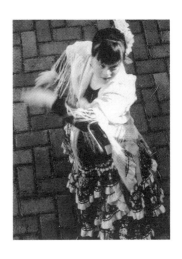

chapter 8

'A DIFFERENT WAY OF LOOKING'

'Having a different way of looking at things is something we should all embrace.'
(David Giles, 'The Three Daves', *West Australian*,
26 November 2009)

Justin Marshall started his public career in 1999 as a year twelve schoolboy when he received a writing award for an essay on living with Down syndrome.[129] His mother described it as 'an innocent beginning,' but from that moment, Justin took on a role speaking about having Down syndrome at schools, to training groups and on any number of public panels, including appearances alongside Western Australia's deputy commissioner for police Chris Dawson and burns specialist Dr Fiona Wood ('The Cop, the Doc and Justin'), and with other high profile sports people ('The Runner, Rider, Rower and Retiree') for the International Day of People with Disability in 2007 and 2008. Justin was 'the rower' on the 2008 panel, having won gold medals in adaptive rowing events at the National Rowing Championships in Victoria and Tasmania, and he has also been the WA Disabled Sports Powerlifting Champion four times in a row.[130] Over the last ten years he has delivered literally hundreds of speeches, including one at an international congress in Singapore, and as his mother Margaret Marshall said: 'It's hard to believe that I used to worry about his painfully slow speech development and wonder if he would ever be able to express himself properly!'

Some of Justin's reflections on his life appear at the front of this book.

David Guhl is less articulate than Justin and does not read or write, but he has found ways of expressing himself through dance and art. He is a regular performer with DADAA (Disability in the Arts, Disadvantage in the Arts, Western Australia) and Strutdance, and has made a number of acclaimed appearances with prize-winning dancers and choreographers Sete Tele and Rachel Ogle. As an artist, Dave has had two major exhibitions. His first, *Truly Madly Delightful* in 2008, was a sell-out, with twenty-three of his twenty-eight works sold in the first hour; his second, *The Three Daves*, a joint art exhibition designed to bring together aspects of disability, mental illness and 'normal' life, was equally successful, with the *West Australian*'s art critic Ric Spencer describing Dave Guhl's 'deliriously colourful landscapes' as representing 'the actuality of existence and the possibility of seeing with open eyes.'[131] Dave Guhl has won six art awards, has judged a number of art prizes and has paintings in several public collections including the City of Perth, the Town of Vincent, and the WA Office of Legal Aid. One of his paintings appears on the cover of this book.

People with Down syndrome are doing extraordinary things today. They are also doing ordinary everyday things, and in the light of the history of the past fifty years, that is just as wonderful. A few decades ago, social expectations of people with Down syndrome were minimal, but things have changed. Not all people with Down syndrome are public speakers like Justin, prize-winning artists like David, or hold world records in sporting events like Stephen Donovan, and it is undoubtedly easier to document the outstanding than the ordinary. But today, people with Down syndrome are busy doing perfectly normal things, getting on with their lives. Most need a degree of support, some more than others, but in many ways society is adapting to the task of accommodating difference. In Western Australia people with disabilities have been fortunate in that the government has supported many of the strategies that have brought about changes since the 1970s. Of course there is never enough money, never enough housing, and families have sometimes had to wait an unacceptably long time for help, but over time a shift in understandings about disability has meant real improvement in the lives led by many people with disabilities such as Down syndrome. The Western Australian government's Future Directions 2025 strategy, for example, which will focus on making changes in the areas of 'economic and community foundations', 'participation and contribution' and 'personalised supports and services' for people with disabilities, should continue to raise expectations for the future, improve outcomes and reaffirm the value of providing support.[132] Families can never afford to be complacent but, as the history of disability shows, things do sometimes move forward.

Changes have not been uniformly exciting though. School classrooms remain a battleground for some parents. Improvements in the provision of health services for people with disabilities have had an enormously positive impact on both the length and quality of life for people with Down syndrome, but at the same time, too many examples reveal that some individual medical practitioners are still unable to come to terms with the notion that people with Down syndrome require first class, not second class service. The rate of termination of babies with Down syndrome also suggests that while social acceptance of people born with conditions such as Down syndrome is getting better, there is still deep ambivalence about welcoming disability into individual homes and families.

Also at an individual level, we continue to hear stories which remind us of the legacy of ignorance and stupidity still to be overcome. In a sports story in 2008, the *Sydney Morning Herald* told how New South Wales rugby league star Craig Wing 'was playing for the Roosters against the Bulldogs at the Sydney Football Stadium, [when] a Bulldogs fan screamed, 'F–— you Wing, your sister has Down syndrome.'[133] Wing's response was incredulity. Family is of course beyond the pale when it comes to sledging, a practice which most players accept as a normal if unpleasant aspect of being a high profile sporting personality. But the story underlines continuing division within society about Down syndrome and disability more generally. The ugliness of the language is matched only by the ugliness of the sentiments it represents. Clearly there is a sector of society, and not just confined to football fans, which still considers having a family member with a disability such as Down syndrome to be shameful.

Over the past fifty years we have seen the lives of people with disabilities change almost beyond recognition as expectations of their capacities have grown but it seems clear that society itself has to change a little more to keep up with this new reality. One mother said, 'I think it's really society that has to adapt, not the kids, because in reality they have only a certain amount of room to move and then it's us that have to flex.'[134] The more that people with Down syndrome and other disabilities are included in the community, the more visible they become, the greater the chance that society itself can 'flex' to continue to accommodate 'difference' as normality. There is still a way to go.

Within the family, what is it like to live with Down syndrome? Families were quick to realise that living with a difference was not as fearful as they had first imagined. At the very least, they have had to look at decision-making more carefully and be more astute about forward planning but they have also learnt to adapt, stretch and grow. Not all of this is painful! It generally doesn't take long from the moment when families learn of their new member's disability and fear they have said goodbye to life as they know it, to realise that life does go on, if in a slightly unexpected direction. Nothing says it better than Emily Perl Kingsley's wonderful metaphor of having a child with a disability — after enthusiastically preparing for a trip to Italy, instead you find yourself arriving in Holland.[135] Not at all where you planned to be but not such a bad place after the initial shock: just different!

Given positive expectations, there is little reason for opportunities and life chances to close off after a child with a disability is born, and sometimes they can even be enhanced. With Stephen Donovan travelling the world to international swimming competitions, for example, his family has had the opportunity to go with him to Portugal, Ireland, Taiwan and beyond. Our family packed up and went to live in the United States for six months with no qualms about Maddie's capacity to cope. Other families have spent sabbaticals in Italy, travelled to the Himalayas, or plan to walk the Kokoda track. These aspirations may not be realistic for all people with Down syndrome — they might be unrealistic for some people without Down syndrome too — but high expectations are everything.

The emotional impact of sharing your life with a family member with Down syndrome is far more complicated, far more profound than this, and conveying what it is like is as challenging as trying to explain to a sceptical childless friend the virtues of having children. You soon find yourself embarrassed by your own hyperbole, and convinced they are thinking, 'Well she would say that, wouldn't she!' One mother, who often speaks publicly about her son with Down syndrome, experiences the same difficulty when dealing with this topic, and told me, tongue-in-cheek, that she has to try hard to avoid the 'every home should have one' approach. It's not an experience either of us sought but it has changed and enriched both of us beyond measure, and perhaps beyond explanation.

For people with Down syndrome themselves, what it means to live with Down syndrome seems equally hard to explain — it was generally a non-issue, or at least not one they thought worth discussing. Jeremy Young suggested that having diabetes was a much more significant factor in his life. Rachel Kingston assured me that though she had once had Down syndrome, she no longer did, though her parents hadn't realised this yet. Justin Marshall wrote that people with Down syndrome are normal and should be treated so,[136] and Eloise Hartley said exactly the same thing. Ellen Wentworth was adamant that having Down syndrome meant nothing to her at all.

My own daughter Maddie knows she has Down syndrome, but for her, all that means is that she occasionally needs a little more support than her sisters. In fact, that is how she views all her friends with disabilities: as regular people who sometimes need just that little bit of extra help to get to the same place as everyone else. It's really just a question of a different way of looking.

NOTES

Introduction

1 House of Representatives, *Hansard*, 15 November 1979, pp. 3146–7, Mr John Martyr, Member for Swan; *Perth Weekend News*, 17 November 1979; typescript (from Mrs Doris Martyr), 'An Episode of Innocence', in author's possession.

2 'Transplant "pioneer" with Down's syndrome dies', *CNN News*, 25 May 1997, http://cgi.cnn.com/US/9705/25/disabled.transplant (accessed 26 March 2008).

3 Kathy Evans, *Tuesday's Child*, Bantam, Sydney, 2007, p. 83.

4 Brian Stratford, *Down's Syndrome: Past, Present and Future*, Penguin Books, London, 1989, pp. 154–5.

5 Patricia E. Bauer, 'Public man, private father', News and commentary on disability issues, 4 June 2007, http://www.patriciaebauer.com/2007/06/04/public-man-private-father-29 (accessed 1 April 2008).

6 Suzanna Andrews, 'Arthur Miller's Missing Act', *Vanity Fair*, September 2007, http://www.vanityfair.com/fame/features/2007/09/miller200709 (accessed 1 April 2008).

7 Some of my earlier views on this project and its offshoots are discussed in Jan Gothard, 'Beyond the myths: representing people with Down syndrome', in Monica Cuskelly, Anne Jobling and Susan Buckley (eds), *Down Syndrome: Across the Life Span*, London and Philadelphia, 2002, pp. 2–15.

8 Jan Walmsley, 'Life History Interviews with People with Learning Disabilities', *Oral History*, Spring 1995, p. 72.

9 I have discussed these issues more extensively in Jan Gothard, 'Oral history, ethics, intellectual disability and empowerment: an inside perspective' in Cathie Clement (ed.), *Studies in Western Australian History: Ethics and the Practice of History*, vol. 26, 2010.

10 The intimacy of the subjects addressed in interviews, and the fact that they related to intensely private feelings, meant that with the agreement of the participants, all interview material in this book is used anonymously. Yet this decision has ethical implications. At a symposium at La Trobe University in Melbourne in December 2007, where a number of formerly institutionalised people with intellectual disabilities spoke out about their hidden lives behind the walls of places such as Kew Cottages, discussants were vehement about the need both to have their voices heard and to be named. If conducting this project again, I would ask my informants with Down syndrome to permit me to use their real names.

11 Ann Curthoys, 'History and reminiscence: writing about the anti-Vietnam-War movement', in Susan Magarey with Caroline Guerin and Paula Hamilton (eds), *Writing Lives: Feminist Biography and Autobiography*, Australian Feminist Studies Publications, Adelaide, 1992, p. 118.

12 Karen Hirsch, 'Culture and disability: The role of oral history', in Robert Perks and Alistair Thomson, *The Oral History Reader*, London and New York, 1998, p. 220.

13 Brian Stratford, *Down's Syndrome,* p. 106.

14 Tim Booth and Wendy Booth, 'Sounds of silence: narrative research with inarticulate subjects', *Disability and Society,* vol. 11, no. 1, 1996; Mark Rapley, *The Social Construction of Intellectual Disability,* Cambridge University Press, New York, 2004.

Chapter 1

15 Fay Weldon, *Darcy's Utopia,* Collins, London, 1990, p. 140.

16 The APGAR test is an analysis of a baby's physical condition given immediately after birth.

17 Most general books on Down syndrome list these features and their implications. See for example, Karen Stray-Gundersen, *Babies with Down Syndrome: A New Parents' Guide,* Woodbine House, Bethesda MD, 1995, second edition, pp. 17–21.

18 N. Breheny, P. O'Leary, J. Dickinson, C. Bower, J. Goldblatt, B. Hewitt, A. Murch and R. Stock, *Statewide evaluation of first trimester screening for Down syndrome and other fetal anomalies in Western Australia,* Genomics Occasional Paper 5, Prenatal Diagnosis Committee, Department of Health, Western Australia, 2005, p. 3.

19 Brian Stratford, *Down's Syndrome,* appendix, 'The biological basis of Down's Syndrome', pp. 165–6.

20 'Kay's story', Bush Telegraph. A Newsletter from your Mid West Local Area Coordination Team, Disability Services Commission, October 2009, p.1.

21 For more information, see for example, Mark Selikowitz, *Down Syndrome: The Facts,* third edition, Oxford University Press, 2008; Brian Stratford, *Down's Syndrome,* p. 89, and appendix, pp. 156–79.

22 Jon Henley, 'Children like Grace', *The Guardian,* 4 October 2007, http://www.guardian.co.uk/society/2007/oct/04/socialexclusion. medicineandhealth (accessed 1 April 2008).

23 Nigel Lawson, 'All you need is life', *Spectator,* 17 June 1995, reprinted *Sydney Morning Herald,* 19 June 1995.

24 Jerome Lejeune identified trisomy in 1959.

25 John Langdon Down, 1866.

26 Clare Campbell, 'The joy and pain of raising our Down's baby', *Daily Mail,* 19 May 2006, http://www.dailymail.co.uk/pages/live/femail/article. html?in_article_id=386926&in_page_id=1879 (accessed 4 April 2008).

Chapter 2

27 Peter Singer, *Practical Ethics,* 2nd edition, Cambridge University Press, 1993, p. 188.

28 See Charles Fox, 'Debating Deinstitutionalisation: The Fire at Kew Cottages in 1996 and the Idea of Community', *Journal of the Australian Society of the History of Medicine, Health and History,* Deinstitutionalisation, Special Issue, vol. 5, no. 2, 2003, p. 56.

29 Corinne Manning, *Bye-Bye Charlie: Stories from the Vanishing World of Kew Cottages,* UNSW Press, Sydney, 2008, pp. 28–50.

30 Leonie Stella, 'Normalisation and Beyond: Public sector residential care 1965–1990', in E. Cocks, C. Fox, M. Brogan and M. Lee (eds), *Under Blue Skies: The Social Construction of Intellectual Disability in Western Australia*, Edith Cowan University, 1996, p. 96.

31 Christina Gillgren, ' "Once a defective, always a defective": Public sector residential care 1900–1965', in Cocks, Fox, Brogan and Lee (eds), *Under Blue Skies*, pp. 84–5.

32 Name withheld.

33 See IDSC for Life website, http://idscforlife.wordpress.com (accessed 30 June 2010).

34 GovTrack.us, 'S. 1810 [110th Congress 2007–2008]: Prenatally and Postnatally Diagnosed Conditions Awareness Act', *GovTrack.us* (database of federal legislation), http://www.govtrack.us/congress/bill. xpd?bill=s110-1810 (accessed 7 October 2008).

35 Senator Ted Kennedy, cited in 'Saving Nathan's Bill might reduce abortion of Down syndrome babies', Disabled Rights Alliance, 21 Nov 2007, http://groups.google.com.au/group/DISABLED-RIGHTS-ALLIANCE/ browse_thread/thread/726cb136ab46f3c5 (accessed 7 October 2008).

36 Leah Merton, Senior Scientist, Western Diagnostic Pathology to author, 15 October 2008; see also P. O'Leary, N. Breheny, G. Reid, T. Charles and J. Emery, 'Regional variations in prenatal screening across Australia: Stepping towards a national policy framework', *Australian and New Zealand Journal of Obstetrics and Gynaecology*, 2006, vol. 46, no. 5, pp. 427–32.

37 P. O'Leary et al., 'Regional variations in prenatal screening across Australia', p. 42, table 1.

38 Western Diagnostic Pathology, *Understanding First Trimester Pregnancy Screening: Information for Patients*, n.d.

39 See Sam Solomon, 'New prenatal screening guidelines spark row', *National Review of Medicine*, Canada, vol. 4, no. 4, 28 Feb 2007.

40 Melinda Tankard Reist (in *Defiant Birth: Women who resisted medical eugenics*, Spinifex Press, North Melbourne, 2006, pp. 13–16) discusses the issue of the right not to know. The book also deals with other issues discussed in this chapter.

41 See Sam Solomon, 'New prenatal screening guidelines spark row'.

42 See for example, Sylvie St-Jacques, Sonya Grenier, Marc Charland, Jean-Claude Forest, Francois Rousseau and France Légaré, 'Decisional needs assessment regarding Down syndrome prenatal testing: a systematic review of the perceptions of women, their partners and health professionals', *Prenatal Diagnosis*, 2008, vol. 28, no. 16, pp. 1183–203, which reviews thirty-two separate studies of this issue.

43 Melinda Tankard Reist, *Defiant Birth*, p. 133.

44 S. Leonard, C. Bower, B. Petterson and H. Leonard, 'Survival of infants born with Down's syndrome: 1980–96', *Paediatrics and Perinatal Epidemiology*, 2000, vol. 14, pp. 163–71.

45 'Down syndrome kids have much to contribute: mums', *West Australian*, 17 May 2008.

46 Jackie Softly, former executive officer, DSAWA.

47 Warwick J. Neville and Buddhima Lokuge, 'Wrongful life claims: dignity, disability and "a line in the sand"', *Medical Journal of Australia*, 20 November 2006, vol. 185, no. 10, pp. 558–60.

48 Dave Reynolds, 'Proposal Would Keep People From Filing "Wrongful Birth" Lawsuits', *Inclusion Daily Express,* 15 January 2002, http://www.inclusiondaily.com/news/advocacy/wrongfulbirths.htm (accessed 1 July 2010).

49 Kate Hagan, 'Hospital "should have told" of Down's risk', *The Age*, online, 19 September 2009.

50 See Melinda Tankard Reist, *Defiant Birth*, pp. 13–16, on 'the right not to know'.

51 See Elizabeth De Souza, Jane Halliday, Annabelle Chan, Carol Bower and Joan K. Morris, 'Recurrence risks for trisomies 13, 18, and 21', *American Journal of Medical Genetics*, Part A, vol. 149A, pp. 2716–22.

52 Michael Bérubé, 'We still don't know what "normal" really is', *The Globe and Mail*, 7 March 2007, http://www.theglobeandmail.com/life/article746031. ece (accessed 29 June 2010).

53 'Down's births: How BBC misread the evidence', *The Guardian*, 29 November 2008, http://www.guardian.co.uk/commentisfree/2008/ nov/29/downs-syndrome-bbc (accessed 26 June 2010).

54 'Down's Syndrome Live Births in England and Wales (1989–2006)', National Down Syndrome Cytogenetic Register, Wolfson Institute of Preventive Medicine, http://www.wolfson.qmul.ac.uk/ndscr/update/livebirths.html (accessed 26 June 2010; page updated 25 November 2009).

Chapter 3

55 This discriminatory practice is permitted to the government's migration officers under the Commonwealth's 1992 *Disability Discrimination Act*, which explicitly exempts the Migration Act and those enforcing it from its provisions.

56 Statistics from IDEA Database, Telethon Institute for Child Health Research, Perth, Western Australia, supplied by Jenny Bourke, TICHR.

57 Karen Stray-Gundersen, *Babies with Down Syndrome,* p. 65.

58 See Seonaid Leonard et al., 'Survival of infants born with Down's syndrome', pp. 163–71.

59 ibid., p. 163.

60 Dr Luigi D'Orsogna, interview with Jan Gothard, 28 August 2008.

61 Karen Stray-Gundersen, *Babies with Down Syndrome*, pp. 69–70.

62 ibid., p. 79.

63 Orthopaedic problems, including atlanto-axial instability, or excessive movement between the two upper vertebrae, can occur in children with Down syndrome.

64 Seonaid Leonard et al., 'Survival of infants born with Down's syndrome', pp. 167–9.

65 Email, Dr Cathie Clement to Jan Gothard, 31 July 2010.

66 Alzheimer's Australia, *Living with Dementia: Down syndrome and Alzheimer's disease*, Help Sheet, Alzheimer's Australia, 2005.

67 ibid.
68 Human Rights and Equal Opportunity Commission Mailing List, Disability Rights Update, 7 February 2007.
69 Down's Syndrome Association of UK, 'He'll never join the army', Report, 1998.

Chapter 4

70 The name was officially changed to the Down Syndrome Association of Western Australia (Inc.) on 12 November 1996. The business name — Down Syndrome WA — was registered on 4 January 2008 but the Association remains the Down Syndrome Association of Western Australia (Inc.) and I refer to it as DSAWA throughout this book.
71 Most of this information comes from Charlie Fox, 'Parents' Groups in the 1950s', unpublished referenced manuscript, 2007, p. 4, in author's possession.
72 Charlie Fox, 'Parents' Groups in the 1950s', pp. 5–7. The SLCG was responsible for Irrabeena as an assessment and treatment centre until 1964, at which point responsibility was assumed by the state's Mental Health Services. Irrabeena then formed the basis of the department's Division of the Intellectually Handicapped. See A.S. Ellis, *Eloquent Testimony: The Story of the Mental Health Services in Western Australia 1830–1975*, UWA Press, Nedlands, 1984, pp. 156–7.
73 The name Slow Learning Children's Group (SLCG) was changed to Activ Foundation Inc. in 1986; Activ, http://www.activ.asn.au (accessed 1 July 2010).
74 Charlie Fox, 'Parents' Groups in the 1950s', p. 9.
75 ibid., p. 11.
76 Minutes of meeting of parents interested in forming an organisation, 11 July 1951, cited in Charlie Fox, 'Parents' Groups in the 1950s', p. 13.
77 Leonie Stella, 'Normalisation and beyond: Public Sector Residential Care 1965–1990', in Cocks, Fox, Brogan and Lee (eds), *Under Blue Skies*, p. 96.
78 ibid., p. 93.
79 ibid., ch. 3.
80 As occurs in this sentence, real names are used in the text where they refer to the history of the DSAWA as these names are already in the public domain by way of early minutes, etc. Unless otherwise indicated, all material in this section comes from interviews conducted for this project.
81 Interview, Cathy Donovan, Executive Officer, DSAWA; DSAWA website, http://www.dsawa.asn.au (accessed 1 July 2010); DSAWA Organisational Timeline, email Jackie Softly to Jan Gothard, 2 June 2008.
82 Women and Newborn Health Service, *Report of the Birth Defects Registry of Western Australia 1980–2006*, King Edward Memorial Hospital, November 2007, p. 19.
83 C. Bower et al., *Report of the Birth Defects Registry of Western Australia, 1980–2008*, King Edward Memorial Hospital, Dec 2009, p. 2.
84 Women and Newborn Health Service, *Report of the Birth Defects Registry of Western Australia 1980–2006*, p. 22.

85 See 'History of disability services', DSC website, http://www.disability.
   wa.gov.au (accessed 1 July 2010); see also Leonie Stella, 'Normalisation and
   beyond: Public Sector Residential Care 1965–1990', in Cocks, Fox, Brogan
   and Lee (eds), *Under Blue Skies*, ch. 3 for a detailed account of this and other
   associated shifts.
86 See 'History of disability services', http://www.disability.wa.gov.au
   (accessed 1 July 2010).
87 Name withheld.
88 ibid.
89 ibid.

Chapter 5

90 Individual submission, Department of Education and Training, *Pathways to
   the Future: A Report of the Review of Educational Services for Students with
   Disabilities in Government Schools*, East Perth, 2004, p. 19.
91 Kylie Carman-Brown and Charlie Fox, 'Doctors, Psychologists and
   Educators: The Professions and Intellectual Disability', in Cocks, Fox,
   Brogan and Lee (eds), *Under Blue Skies,* p. 234.
92 *Education in Western Australia*: *Report of the Committee of Inquiry appointed
   by the Minister for Education in Western Australia*, under the chairmanship
   of Mr K. E. Beazley, AO, Perth, March 1984, pp. 302–3.
93 ibid., pp. 35, 299.
94 *The Education of Students with Disabilities and Specific Learning Difficulties*,
   Report of the Ministerial Taskforce, Chaired by Ruth Shean for the
   Minister for Education, Western Australia, Perth, June 1993, p. 180.
95 The capacity of children with Down syndrome to acquire early literacy
   skills and the dividends this pays in terms of later education has been well
   researched and documented through the work of Professor Sue Buckley,
   University of Portsmouth and Down Syndrome Education International, in
   the United Kingdom.
96 DISTAR (Direct Instruction System for Teaching Arithmetic and Reading)
   is a very closely structured direct instruction system for teaching reading
   and numeracy to children. It has been particularly used for children at
   educational risk.
97 Employment, Workplace Relations and Education References Committee,
   Education of Students with Disabilities, Senate Report, December 2002,
   p. 34.
98 ibid., p. xxii.

Chapter 6

99 Disability WA (the website of the Disability Services Commission),
   'Alternatives to Employment, Post School Options and Recreation',
   http://www.disability.wa.gov.au/serviceproviders/guidelinespolicies/
   employmentalternatives2.html (accessed 1 August 2010).
100 Charlie Fox, 'Parents' groups in the 1950s', p. 5.
101 ibid., p. 6.
102 ibid., p. 12.

103 ibid., p. 13.

104 ibid., p. 13.

105 Margaret Hamilton, *EDGE Employment Solutions: Work in Progress – 21 years of placing and supporting people with disabilities in open employment*, Greenwood, Western Australia, 2005, pp. 9–10.

106 *Disability Services Census 2007*, Dept of Families, Housing, Community Services and Indigenous Affairs, Canberra, 2008, section 6.4.1, http://www.fahcsia.gov.au/sa/disability/pubs/policy/Documents/services_census07 (accessed 1 August 2010).

107 ibid., section 4.5.

108 ibid., section 6.4.2.

109 Disability in the Arts, Disadvantage in the Arts, Western Australia.

110 See Susan Brady, John Britton & Sonia Grover, *The Sterilisation of Girls and Young Women in Australia: issues and progress*, A Report jointly commissioned by the Sex Discrimination Commissioner and the Disability Discrimination Commissioner at the Australian Human Rights Commission, 2001, ch. 2; and Susan Brady and Sonia Grover, *The sterilisation of girls and young women in Australia: A a legal, medical and social context*, Human Rights and Equal Opportunity Commission, Disability Discrimination Commissioner, Sydney, 1997.

111 Name withheld.

Chapter 7

112 Independent Living, Canada, http://www.ilcanada.ca/article/home-125. asp (accessed 3 February 2009).

113 Report of Parent Meeting called by the University Class Parent Group of the Slow Learning children, 13 August 1951, in Activ Foundation Archives. Cited in Charlie Fox, 'Parents' Groups in the 1950s'.

114 Christina Gillgren, '"Once a Defective, always a Defective": Public Sector Residential Care 1900–1965', in Cocks, Fox, Brogan and Lee (eds), *Under Blue Skies*, pp. 72–3, 84–6.

115 Kathleen Rhodes, 'Catholic University Honors Popular Teacher Who Killed Her Baby', CNSNews.com, Thursday 27 January 2005, http://97.74.65.51/readArticle.aspx?ARTID=9807 (accessed 18 January 2010).

116 Christina Gillgren, '"Once a Defective, always a Defective": Public Sector Residential Care 1900–1965', in Cocks, Fox, Brogan and Lee (eds), *Under Blue Skies*, p. 87.

117 Leonie Stella, 'Normalisation and beyond: Public Sector Residential Care 1965–1990', in Cocks, Fox, Brogan and Lee (eds) *Under Blue Skies*, ch. 3.

118 Disability Services Commission, WA, 'Community Living Initiative', http://www.disability.wa.gov.au/forindividuals/clivinginitiative.html (accessed 8 June 2010).

119 See 'Independence', *The Diary*, DSAWA, July 2010, p. 18.

120 This information comes from personal conversations with staff at the Western Australian Department of Corrective Services, April 2009; there

are no statistics available to corroborate this empirically in Western Australia.

121 Compic images are simple drawings, called pictographs, designed to convey information without the need for the written or spoken word. The system was developed in Australia and is a useful resource for people with communication or learning difficulties.

122 Department of Housing and Works; formerly Homes West; now Department of Housing.

123 See Charlie Fox, 'Debating Deinstitutionalisation', for a discussion of different understandings of communities and their roles in deinstitutionalisation.

124 Telephone conversation, Angie Godden, Mid West Community Living Association, 16 March 2009.

125 Disability Services Commission, WA, 'Community Living Initiative', http://www.disability.wa.gov.au/forindividuals/clivinginitiative.html (accessed 8 June 2010).

126 Al Etmanski with Jack Collins and Vicki Cammack, *Safe and Secure: Six Steps to Creating a Good Life for People with Disabilities*, Planned Lifetime Advocacy Network (PLAN), Western Australian edition, 2008.

127 http://pin0.businesscatalyst.com/index.htm (accessed 10 June 2010).

128 Charlie Fox, 'Debating Deinstitutionalisation', p. 44. See also Christine Bigby, 'Known well by no-one: trends in the informal social networks of middle-aged and older people with intellectual disability five years after moving to the community', *Journal of Intellectual and Developmental Disability*, 2008, vol. 33, no. 2, pp. 148–57.

Chapter 8

129 *Christchurch Grammar School Chronicle*, June 1999, p. 26.

130 *Mosman Cottesloe Post*, 30 March 2002; *West Australian*, n.d., 2004; *The Westie*, September 2006.

131 *West Australian*, 26 November 2009; *The Three Daves*, catalogue, 2009.

132 Future Directions 2025, http://www.disability.wa.gov.au/dsc/corpdocuments/countmeindfd/aboutdfd.html (accessed 31 Aug 2010).

133 *Sydney Morning Herald*, 16 July 2008.

134 Diana Foster interview.

135 Emily Perl Kingsley, *Welcome to Holland*, 1987, http://www.our-kids.org/Archives/Holland.html (accessed 31 August 2010).

136 *Christchurch Grammar School Chronicle*, June 1999, p. 26.

INDEX

First published 2011 by
FREMANTLE PRESS
25 Quarry Street, Fremantle 6160
(PO Box 158, North Fremantle 6159)
Western Australia
www.fremantlepress.com.au

Editor Janet Blagg
Cover Design Allyson Crimp
Printed by Everbest Printing Company Pty Ltd, China

National Library of Australia
Cataloguing-in-Publication entry (pbk)

Gothard, Janice.

Greater expectations : living with Down syndrome in the
 twenty-first century / by Jan Gothard.

1st ed.

ISBN 9781921361777 (pbk.)

Down syndrome--Social aspects.
 People with mental disabilities--Social aspects.
 People with mental disabilities--Australia--Social conditions.
 Down syndrome.

362.196858842

Publication of this title was assisted by the Commonwealth Government
through the Australia Council, its arts funding and advisory body.